THE PHYSICIAN'S ASSOCIATE

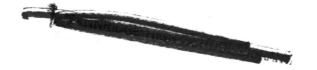

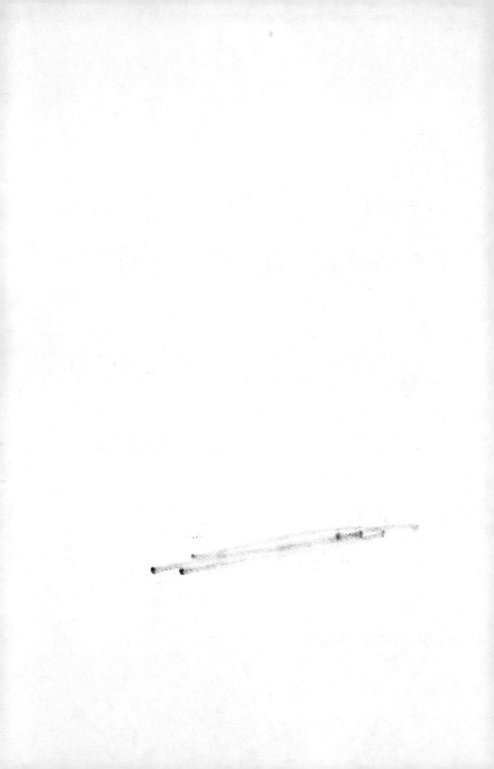

THE Physician's Associate

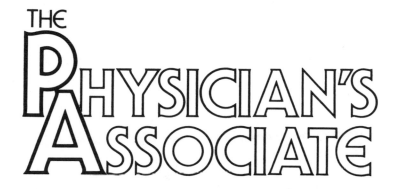

A NEW CAREER IN HEALTH CARE

Ann Cavallaro

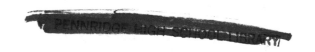

ELSEVIER/NELSON BOOKS
New York

Library of Congress Cataloging in Publication Data

Cavallaro, Ann.
   The physician's associate: a new career in health care

   Includes index.
   I. Physicians' assistants—Vocational guidance.
I. Title.
R697.P45C38   610.69'53   78–2369
ISBN 0–525–66598–6

Published in the United States by Elsevier/Nelson Books, a division of Elsevier-Dutton Publishing Company, Inc., New York. Published simultaneously in Don Mills, Ontario, by Thomas Nelson and Sons (Canada) Limited.
Printed in the U.S.A.
10 9 8 7 6 5 4 3 2

CONTENTS

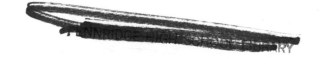

AUTHOR'S NOTE

This book presents a spectrum of ideas and facts concerning a relative newcomer to health occupations—the physician's associate. It is addressed to several categories of readers:

1. The high-school junior or senior considering a health career.

2. The junior-college or community-college student contemplating transfer into a senior-college program.

3. The student now attending college (or on leave of absence) who seeks a change in curriculum, or the college graduate desiring a health profession that can be learned, if not mastered, in a period of two years or less.

4. The adult engaged in a patient-care service who wishes to upgrade his or her knowledge, skills, and career status.

I was fortunate in being allowed to spend entire days with physicians' associates at their jobs. This has given me a vivid and immediate "feel" for the subject, as well as an appreciation of the impressive work being performed.

Any study such as this one, which spells out tuition costs, educational fees, and salaries, runs the risk of courting inaccuracies, since prices change continuously. The reader, I am sure, will understand why some of the costs he encounters do not agree with mine.

I am grateful to all persons named or designated by names other than their own. Without them there would be no book.

A.C.

THE PHYSICIAN'S ASSOCIATE

1

A DAY IN THE LIFE OF A PHYSICIAN'S ASSOCIATE

Geoffrey Francoeur

"Friday is relatively light," explains Geoffrey Francoeur. "We're kept busy, but it's nothing like Monday or Tuesday. On a typical Monday, I see fifteen to twenty patients. And up to twenty-five emergencies."

Is this man who sees patients and treats emergencies a doctor? Not quite. He belongs to the newest and most exciting branch of medical service—physicians' associates.

Geoffrey's job is to perform routine medical examinations, thus speeding up treatment and increasing the efficiency of medical services in the hospital. What does all this involve? Well, let's spend a day with Geoffrey and see for ourselves.

He arrives at the veteran's hospital where he is employed at eight in the morning, dons a white coat, checks his equipment, and consults his calendar. Does he need to check test results with the hospital laboratory? Did he promise to report findings to a patient? Has anything unusual been scheduled by the administration? He answers these and other questions to himself and makes a mental plan for his day. Then he reviews the notes he has jotted down for the weekly staff meeting, during which suggestions and procedures are discussed. Memory refreshed, he heads for his meeting.

By the time the meeting is over—it seldom runs longer than half an hour—the reception corridor bulges with men and a few women, seated on multicolored molded-plastic chairs. These are the members of the outpatient division of the Veteran's Administration hospital where Geoffrey works.

The medical staff of the division consists of five physicians, each with his own small office, nurses, clerks, and Geoffrey. Clinic-fashion, each patient is seen by the first available physician, not necessarily the one who had previously treated him or given him this date to return. A doctor may indicate on the record, however, that the patient is to return to him. (Geoffrey, too, has this choice.)

The patient, returning or new, first sees the evaluation clerk, explains his problem, and shows his evaluation card. The clerk adds a brief statement to the record and places it in a file accessible to all the doctors. If the patient is new or has not been tested lately, urinalysis and blood tests are done routinely, as well as a chest X ray and electrocardiograph. These results are then incorporated into the record, and the patient is told to be seated, to wait until Geoffrey or one of the doctors is free.

As in most free clinics, there is usually a long wait for medical attention. Geoffrey feels strongly that this should be changed. "We can't see all thirty people at eight A.M.," he objects. "It would be easier on the patients if we gave approximate-time appointments. But that would involve more bookkeeping."

Geoffrey's first patient, a cheerful Oriental-American in his forties, complains of a lingering sore throat. He speaks without hoarseness and reports no other difficulties; his breathing and temperature are normal.

Geoffrey takes a throat culture and tells the patient he will be contacted by telephone as soon as the results come in from the hospital laboratory, normally within a day. He explains that the infection will probably disappear on its own, but he is concerned about the remote possibility of a hemolytic streptococcus infection (Type A) which, if untreated, might affect the kidneys.

Before seeing a second patient, Geoffrey carefully enters his findings into the record and places it in the evaluation clerk's office for filing. He returns with the record of the next patient, a sixty-eight-year-old veteran, who is here for the second time with a complaint of lingering backache. In every instance the medical record and evaluation sheet are painstakingly read before the patient is admitted to the examination room.

This patient suffered a fall on the ice six months earlier but did not feel severe pain at that time or seek medical assistance, assuming his discomfort would "go away." X rays taken at the time of his first visit are negative—that is, they do not reveal anything out of order.

Geoffrey performs a careful, twenty-five minute, essentially orthopedic examination, questioning the patient concerning his backache—does it bother him while bending, twisting, turning, raising arms and legs, rising on toes, and other normal motions? The patient appears very anxious, fearing that if he can no longer perform what he calls "light-duty work," he will not be able to continue living in the Salvation Army shelter and will be forced to become a state welfare charge.

He leaves the clinic with prescriptions for a muscle relaxant and an analgesic, together with careful and simply phrased instructions for their use. Geoffrey also makes an appointment for him with the orthopedic clinic in approximately ten days.

While entering his findings into the record, Geoffrey tells one of the nurses that he wishes dictating machines were available. "There are some good reasons for not using them in this unit," he admits. "It ties up the record. Sometimes a patient is referred to another department there and then. Or a hospital bed is needed at once. I can see that the record must be available immediately, not waiting its turn in the typing pool. But it would sure save a lot of time to *talk* the record instead of having to write it. . . ."

The next patient, a fifty-one-year-old male, also presents an orthopedic problem triggered by a fall. X rays had been taken the week before. Geoffrey consults these (still on file within the unit, rather than in the X-ray library on another floor of the hospital) and discusses them with his patient. There is some bone separation in the shoulder, which might require surgery. Geoffrey points out the asymmetry visible to the naked eye. He instructs the patient in the use of a wide arm sling to inactivate the shoulder. This patient, too, is referred to the orthopedic outpatient clinic.

Geoffrey's next patient, a fifty-five-year-old man, has been seen several times. Today he comes in complaining of a hernia. He is a difficult patient, given to jabbering disconnectedly about his self-diagnoses, his military history as a parachutist, his long-time defiance of medical recommendations, his contempt for doctors and medicine. "When I had frozen feet in Korea, I didn't bother going to a doctor. I let a broken leg heal itself."

Geoffrey smiles patiently. "It usually will, sir. But I think you're wise to come back for a little help."

Careful questioning reveals that the patient has had difficulty in urinating, that he rises three or four times a night, finds sleep elusive, and has not had a complete health check for five years or longer. He boasts self-consciously about this last fact. "And," he adds proudly, "I still put away two packs of cigarettes a day." Yes, he admits, there *is* occasional hoarseness.

Geoffrey spends nearly forty-five minutes in the actual examination of this patient, whose responses and suggestions continue in a rapid, diffuse rat-a-tat. He assures the patient that there is no hernia. He does, however, have an enlarged prostate. An immediate appointment is made with the urology clinic, which Geoffrey urges the patient to keep. He also urges an annual physical examination—and utters the now standard warning about prolonged cigarette smoking, which produces a grin of absolute disbelief. "Look, I started smoking at age ten—I shoulda been dead long ago, Doc."

Lunch for Geoffrey is at no specific time. The patient session must be terminated at a logical point and the record completed and returned to the evaluation clerk's office. Geoffrey, like most VA employees, has lunch in the excellent cafeteria within the installation (there is also a canteen with push-button food and beverages). "Oh no, I wouldn't think of going off the grounds for lunch," he says in answer to a friend's suggestion. "I'm sure I'd never find my parking place again—or any other parking place."

Waiting, when he returns to his office, is a patient he has requested specifically to see—the first and only female of the day, a World War II WAC. She was Geoffrey's patient eight days earlier, when he removed a sebaceous cyst from her back and prescribed antibiotics. He now checks the healing, dresses the wound, and advises the patient to continue the medication until the original prescription is exhausted.

Since this is a veteran's hospital, it is obvious why Geoffrey sees so many men and so few women, and why most of his patients are elderly. "It took a little getting used to," he says. "At my last job [in the emergency room of a Connecticut hospital], I had every kind of patient—and lots of kids."

A Veteran's Administration hospital does not offer maternity, pediatric, or a whole range of other services obtainable at general hospitals. Many younger servicemen, gainfully employed and covered by a variety of health-insurance plans, prefer to see private physicians and use the facilities of voluntary hospitals. Ex-servicewomen are still relatively few in number.

The next patient, an eighty-year-old man, shuffles in apologetically, speaking an accented, halting English; he seems very confused. He was seen a few days before by one of the physicians in the unit and was given medication and an appointment to the urological clinic. Nevertheless, he returns complaining of his symptoms and clutching his blue ID card and the appointment slip.

Geoffrey feels he should not intervene in the treatment being undertaken on behalf of this patient by a specialized department. He explains this carefully to the patient, urges him to continue the medication, and to keep his appointment. The old gentleman shuffles off, still confused, no doubt disappointed.

A forty-six-year-old veteran comes in, led by his very determined wife, a hospital employee in uniform. She states that she had to force her husband to come, so reluctant was he to seek advice. "It's only that I get these headaches," he explains. "Mostly here in front, worse on the left side, maybe."

"Tell him about the nosebleeds," she orders.

"Well, they stopped. I don't get them no more."

"And the time your eye popped out—right from its socket—"

He shrugs, embarrassed. "That was only once."

"And they're always bloodshot—"

"Heck, take a good look—everybody's eyes are bloodshot."

But her recital of symptoms outlasts his protests, and he sheepishly yields. Since the patient is in for the first time, routine X rays and tests are made available to

Geoffrey. Those, plus his own calm, unhurried questions, construct a picture of a man whose body is flashing
danger signals.

After taking an exhaustive medical history, Geoffrey
performs a thorough head-to-toe examination. He literally goes over the patient inch by inch. Eyes, ears, nose,
throat, neck and back muscles, toes, ankles, feet (he
discovers a fungal infection between the patient's toes, of
which the patient and his wife are unaware) are
examined, and all the while the quiet, low-key questions
continue.

Clear, careful explanation and reassurance are Geoffrey's special strengths. He is very good at interpreting
medical facts to patients. His language is simple and
nontechnical, and he withholds nothing. Husband and
wife are told at once that most test results have proved
negative—that is, that nothing has been found to be
wrong. But the eye incident (subconjunctival hemorrhage) and the headaches and nosebleeds might have
been caused by hypertension (high blood pressure), a
problem that calls for immediate corrective measures.
Weight reduction—the patient weighed in at 213
pounds and is hardly five feet seven—is strongly recommended. Rather than attempt piecemeal solutions,
Geoffrey telephones the hypertension clinic of the VA
hospital, only to find it fully booked for three months.

Since the patient is employed and now seems eager
to get on with the treatment, he is urged to go that very
week to the hypertension clinic of a nearby teaching
hospital. Geoffrey finds the clinic does patients more
good than many private physicians can, for it operates an
education program in diet, exercise, principles of nutri-

tion, understanding of hypertension, and health maintenance. Few busy practitioners, however expert, have the time to explain to patients what their condition is and why it needs to be treated. Geoffrey writes out a prescription, and the couple leaves with expressions of relief, gratitude, and promises of future checkups at regular intervals.

When they have departed, Geoffrey takes the X-ray plates to the radiological consultant. "By golly, he *is* fat!" the radiologist bellows on viewing the plates.

So evenly larded is the patient's middle that the rib cage appears incomplete.

Is Geoffrey Francoeur practicing medicine? Definitely.

Is he receiving careful supervision? He has access to the services of the chief medical officer, several primary-care physicians, and numerous specialists. His unit head is a door away. His records are immediately available for review.

Is he capable of performing the duties assigned to him, involving patient history, evaluation of examination and tests, simple surgical procedures, a preliminary diagnosis, referral if indicated? He probably handles these more carefully, unhurriedly, and accurately than the average private doctor, who may be overwhelmed by sheer numbers and frequently by massive fatigue.

Do his patients mistakenly believe him to be a physician? In all likelihood, some do; a few called him Doc. There is no attempt to deceive, however. His badge reads "Physician's Assistant." His signature on a prescription is followed by the initials "P.A." and is subject to review by his superior. He is "mister" to the clinic staff.

He is also a pioneer in his chosen career, one of five admitted to the pilot PA training program of a distinguished university—and that in itself brought him a long, long way from his beginnings.

Geoffrey Francoeur is a West Indian black, who, at the time of his admission, had little education beyond high school. From early childhood he had regarded the world of medicine with reverential awe, but he knew that he could not hope to become a doctor. The small Caribbean island where he was born—part of the British Commonwealth—had no university for him to be trained at.

There was little economic opportunity for him. In the primitive economy of his home island, the best he could look forward to was being a trusted house servant or a tourist-hotel flunky.

Geoffrey now admits that he did not exert himself in high school. What could come of it? At an early age he decided that there was only one solution: he must emigrate to England, where life was more promising.

He arrived during a landslide migration of East and West Indians, Pakistanis, and dark-skinned persons from other Commonwealth countries, each with hopes resembling his own. There was frantic competition among the immigrants for the poorest, least desirable jobs.

Britain had not emerged from World War II a rich country. "Austerity" was the slogan, and the dark-skinned immigrant often found himself disliked and blamed for economic woes. To a West Indian without higher education, London offered little more than job hunting and drudgery. After a year and a half in England, Geoffrey went to New England to visit a maternal aunt. He decided to stay.

The United States did offer a living of sorts: window washing, fruit picking, porterage, office cleaning, service as a hospital orderly. Much of the work proved unpleasant, and all of it led exactly nowhere. Besides, hard menial work emptied him of hope and the desire to seek a better life. Geoffrey became afraid of stagnation and regarded the future with desperation.

At that time work was plentiful in defense industries, which offered traineeships in skilled fields with high wages and benefits. But factory work in defense was closed to him, because he was not a citizen, and it would take years to become one. The door was firmly shut.

Geoffrey finally enlisted in the U.S. Navy for a full four-year tour, partly because such a step would lead to American citizenship. Since enlistees were offered a choice of occupation or type of training, he chose the medical corps.

He must have shown aptitude. After training, he became a surgical technician (also called operating-room technician) on a hospital ship, assisting overworked doctors at countless major and minor operations, taking on emergency procedures, and learning much about health care.

He liked the work very much. When his four years of active service were up, Geoffrey decided to use his educational benefits to become a male registered nurse. Nursing, after all, figured prominently in healing. Nurses were respected in the military. They were officers who could rise in rank, responsibility, economic competence. Nursing seemed a desirable—and attainable—next step.

Geoffrey was gratified to be promptly accepted into an associate degree (two-year) course at a large private university in New England. He was already involved in his first semester's work for the R.N. when he learned that a nearby school of medicine was about to inaugurate a physician's associate program.

Things happened quickly. Geoffrey applied, was granted an interview, and quickly assembled his thin credentials. Ten days later he received a letter of acceptance. Quite an achievement for a young black man who had just attained United States citizenship.

At the end of two years' training, Geoffrey went to work in the emergency room of a medium-sized hospital in Connecticut, now his home state. His starting salary was $12,000. Three and a half years later, as an experienced PA, he accepted his present job with the Veteran's Administration at an entering salary of $16,255 and great advancement possibilities.

Geoffrey Francoeur has been educated not to overreach, to be cautious in observing the limits of his training, knowledge, and skills. In doing so, he performs a great health service. He can provide the sorting-out process needed by our undermanned and very specialized physicians. Whether he is the late twentieth century's version of the good old family doctor remains to be seen. But as a team man he can swiftly and efficiently start the patient toward recovery and good health.

Jane Dickinson

Bostonian Jane Dickinson entered Cornell University on graduation from high school without so much as a thought of becoming a physician's associate. She did not aspire to any health career.

"The thought simply hadn't occurred to me," she says. "I majored in history at Cornell, putting off decisions about a career from one year to the next. I don't think students were as career-conscious when I entered college as they are now. You see, jobs were still plentiful all through the sixties. Everywhere you read articles about the dollars-and-cents value of a liberal-arts education.

"The idea was that if you were well-educated you could adapt to any sort of career," she goes on. "And many did. My roommate went to New York right after college and was hired by a publishing house. Another friend—he also majored in English—joined the office of a big utility. They trained him as a systems analyst. By now he's doing very well."

Are such options still available to young graduates? Can college students afford to drift along without career plans?

Jane thinks not. "Now they won't touch unskilled persons who walk in with a nice new B.A. degree. I keep nagging my younger sister—and she's still in high school."

Jane is correct. The economic world has become hostile to the vocationless young, however well educated, adaptable, and able they may be. It is now

imperative that students begin to think of a career while
they are still in high school. Certain careers, such as
engineering and nursing, require an early commitment,
and in all fields, subject preparation is of increasing
importance. With respect to health careers, the competition has become very sharp (Jane calls it "brutal"), and
the standards high.

A bright, energetic blonde, Jane learned of this new
occupation from her brother on his return from Vietnam.
Medical corpsmen were the first to hear about physician's associates, and the first to be sought out by the
new programs that began—experimentally at first—to
train PAs.

As it happened, Jane's brother abandoned his
interest in the new profession. But Jane was fired with
purpose. For the first time in her life—she was already a
college senior—she began to relate to a career, to define
her aspirations, and to see herself as a PA.

First she sent for catalogs describing numerous
programs and studied these carefully. Then she assessed
her own education—and found it wanting. Throughout
her four years in college, having no vocational goal, she
avoided laboratory sciences and mathematics. Her history major did not call for preparation in these disciplin-
es, and she had convinced herself that she didn't like
biology, physics, chemistry, and mathematics.

By the time Jane had decided on her goals, it was
too late to apply for admission immediately after graduation. So Jane spent an interim year studying, taking
courses, filling in what she regarded as her science-math
educational gap. By the time she became an active
candidate, her preparation was quite impressive. Always

a solid student, she found that she continued to perform on a high level even in the disliked areas. Now that she realized the importance of the math-science preparation and its relevance to her career, she no longer found the subjects uninteresting.

Jane read all the catalogs and announcements of every program then in existence. She applied to three and was delighted to be accepted by all of them. She decided on an excellent program about a hundred miles from her home city.

Jane found the PA program difficult but by no means insurmountable. "I guess *challenging* is the right word," she said. The carefully selected students in her class were well prepared for the demands made upon them. The professors, most of them physicians, possessed real conviction concerning the value and need for the program, and they showed almost a personal interest in its success.

"Many doctors do not accept PAs," Jane declares. "Those attached to university centers, especially centers with PA programs, who've seen what can be accomplished—well, they're marvelous. But the average private practitioner with little or no contact . . . some, I'd say, are violently prejudiced."

All graduates of Jane's program promptly procured positions, many in the university medical-center hospitals, two in a methadone-maintenance program, one with a doctor in rural Idaho, one in research. Present salaries, according to Jane and based on figures of her place of employment, range from a beginning $14,000 to a maximum, with experience, of $20,000 to $21,000. (This was in late 1976.)

Jane is delighted with her position as PA in a medical team at a comprehensive health-care center, whose membership is drawn from diverse employee groups. She finds the job varied and interesting, greatly enhancing her own professional growth. "Our in-service education is fantastic," she said.

Jane is one of four PAs assigned by the center to internal-medicine teams. The center also employs a PA in radiology, two in pediatrics, one in "urgent visits" (i.e., serving people who come in without an appointment due to a sudden or emergency problem), and one in miscellaneous specialties. A nurse-midwife with an M.S. degree is assigned to obstetrics.

If Jane can indeed be said to harbor some discontent with her lot, it relates to her professional aspirations. Her training and experience (she joined the health-care center in early 1975) have interested her in becoming a physician. She discussed her ambition to enter medical school with several of the center doctors. They were less than enthusiastic. One conveyed his opinion—not too pleasantly—that the excellent medical education she had received was for the purpose of preparing her to be a PA, not a physician. At about the same time, Jane learned that her two years of PA training at medical school would afford no credits toward the M.D. degree.

Understandably, Jane resents this effort by her colleagues to place a ceiling on her ambitions. Naturally the doctors are insecure at the prospect of dedicated and medically knowledgeable PAs beating on the gates of their own profitable calling.

Jane's day, on paper, runs from nine to five, except on Tuesday, when she reports at twelve thirty and accommodates patients with evening appointments, remaining till nine, nine thirty, or later. She has no weekend work.

In actuality, Jane is at her desk before eight thirty and she seldom leaves at five. There is simply too much to be done—too many patients, too many problems, too little time. She acknowledges the pressures, but does not find them burdensome.

On arrival, Jane consults the night log to learn whether some of her patients have called during her nonworking hours, whether they have been seen by the covering physician, whether any immediate follow-up on her part seems in order.

This will be a particularly heavy week for Jane. One of the three internists on the medical team is on vacation, and she will have to see some of his patients, in addition to her own. She carefully checks the day's schedule and writes out the order in which each scheduled patient's chart (record folder) should be made available.

Requests for prescription renewals, which lie in an accumulated stack, next require attention. Where indicated, she writes out new prescriptions (those to be countersigned by a physician) to be sent to the center's pharmacy. When she does not concur with the request or some reservation prevails, she separates the requests for later telephone explanation or query.

Several records, which she dictated, have been returned by the typing pool and lie on her desk to be corrected, checked, and initialed. Patient records are kept up to date by a combination of longhand entries and transcribed dictation, the latter preferred when the material to be entered into the record is lengthy or involved. Attached to each record is a lined face sheet with a summary of each contact. These sheets are written in columns of cryptic longhand indicating the date of each contact, the nature of the problem, its resolution.

Telephone calls to patients follow. The first involves a patient with a knee injury. Jane's call is a gratifying follow-up—the patient has greatly improved. The second concerns a patient who has undergone tests for a suspected gallbladder condition. Jane is able to tell her that all laboratory tests have been pronounced negative. She reassures the patient, answers numerous questions, suggests diet and antacids to combat the distressing symptoms, and lists foods to be avoided.

Jane's telephoning is interrupted by a messenger from the appointment desk. One of her patients has come in requesting duplication of a medicine that was prescribed for him while he was vacationing in Europe. It is for the treatment of that great plague of tourists, diarrhea. Instructions and label are in Italian.

In a very short time Jane has identified the medication, but it turns out that its manufacture is illegal in the United States. In the process of destroying the hostile bacteria in the digestive tract, the medication also eliminates other benign and necessary bacteria. As a result, yet another medicine is needed to correct the havoc caused by the first. The patient grumbles, not altogether happy or convinced by the explanation, but he accepts the medication Jane substitutes as preferable.

Her second patient of the day is a fifty-year-old woman with a persistent cough, which she has been trying to ignore. Jane examines her ears, nose, throat, chest, and back very carefully. Since this patient has an irregular heartbeat and no other respiratory problems, Jane is reluctant to prescribe a medicine with codeine, which slows the heartbeat. She suggests ordinary cough syrups, gargling, and patience.

The next patient, a young man in his twenties, reports an injury to the knee, resulting from a fall. "My knees buckled," he explains. "Maybe I'm getting too old for sandlot baseball." He grins. "Yes, I know, I know—and my wife keeps telling me to lay off."

He wonders whether removing water from the knee might relieve his symptoms. He has been x-rayed, and nothing has been discovered that would require an orthopedic evaluation, although he wore a brace after the injury. The patient admits that he exhausted himself severely the preceding week, moving his family from one apartment to another by rented truck, without the aid of professional movers.

At first Jane plans to tap the knee. However, after careful examination, she decides against that procedure, which the patient has previously undergone. She finds no serious cartilage damage but feels the fusion far from satisfactory and the tapping now improper. Instead, she suggests he elevate the knee at night and take aspirin at intervals while the pain persists. He is instructed to telephone within a week concerning his progress.

At the end of each patient session, Jane either enters longhand notes into the record or dictates, by telephone switchover, to the typing pool. She is very quick and fluent, keeping these interims to five or ten minutes, in order not to inflict a long wait on her next patient.

One of Jane's "regulars," who has had a slight stroke

and is being seen monthly, arrives for a routine check of her heart condition. She has been taking digitalis and is under strict orders to restrict her food intake and lose weight. Jane regards the woman as a potential diabetic. She weighed in at 170 pounds, badly overweight for a woman only five feet three. She now complains of fatigue, dizziness, assorted aches, shooting pains in the left leg, sore glands, itching surgical scars. Above all, she is finding it impossible to adhere to her 1,000-calorie-a-day diet.

In addition to a very thorough examination, Jane goes into an item-by-item dialogue concerning the patient's daily nutrition. "What do you have for breakfast? . . . How about salt? . . . Do you have a blender? That's wonderful. . . ."

Jane takes and retakes the blood pressure, which is satisfactory. She carefully feels the patient's lymph nodes, asking numerous questions. Because of her anxiety, the patient needs and receives a great deal of supportive encouragement and firm reminders concerning her diet. Jane makes another appointment for the woman and refers her to the center's podiatrist for her sore legs.

The next patient, a bearded man in dungarees who looks much younger than his twenty-nine years, is a long-time diabetic suffering from a cardiac condition. His progress is deemed poor. He came in because he is planning a cross-country automobile trip with a friend and wants to know if it's feasible. Jane is unenthusiastic about his taking so strenuous a journey. She repeats earlier instructions as to rest, medication, and emergencies, and gives him the necessary prescriptions. "He really came to tell me, not to ask me," she says, shaking her head.

A few minutes have to be devoted to a questionnaire from the psychiatric social worker. The center is in the process of conducting research into its own referrals to the mental-health division, with a view to utilizing that department in the most effective way. Jane is participating in the research.

She next telephones one of yesterday's patients. The woman had experienced such a violent headache, diarrhea, and vomiting that she arrived at the center by ambulance in a thoroughly dehydrated condition. She was immediately put on intravenous fluid and allowed to rest at the center for four hours. Jane was on the alert for signs of viral meningitis, but with the intake of fluids the patient's condition improved, and there were no further episodes of vomiting or diarrhea. "I guess it had spent itself," Jane surmised in discharging the woman. Her telephone call corroborates this: the patient reports a normal though tiring day.

Jane is very forthright with patients concerning her status. She introduces herself to a new patient by giving her name, the fact that she is a PA and that she works with the doctors, also indicated by name, in her unit. When called "doctor" she carefully corrects the patient, explaining that she is not a doctor but has had some of a doctor's training in patient care.

A middle-aged woman who suffers from rheumatoid arthritis comes in with a new complaint: warts or "bumps" on her fingers, accompanied by soreness. She has been on gold therapy, with some kidney damage; now she shows a fairly flexible wrist.

Jane calls in one of the doctors on duty in her unit, and after a brief consultation, she advises the patient that the so-called bumps are not warts. "There's a possibility of herpes—a viral skin disease," she says. "I think it would be best to have the dermatologist take a look at you."

Jane tries to get an immediate appointment with the center's dermatologist, but the specialist is not due back from vacation for another three days. The patient is given as early an appointment as possible.

A young mother comes in for a health check. She has no specific symptoms other than lassitude and occasional nausea, an absence of energy, some back pain. She is nursing her infant and working in a day-care center. Jane performs an exhaustive physical examination. She takes a throat culture, arranges for on-the-spot blood work, urinalysis, and chest X ray, and recommends heat, bed rest, swimming, massage as available. The woman is advised that she will be contacted as soon as the reports from the laboratory are made available.

An attractive twenty-eight-year-old black woman with a serious hypertension problem enters, complaining of dizziness and diarrhea. She has been taking extra hormones, and Jane suggests that she stop. Since the blood pressure, measured twice, proves low for her, Jane decreases the blood-pressure medication and suggests adding a small amount of salt to an otherwise salt-free diet. She compliments the patient on her fidelilty to medical instructions. "It's very important to all of us," she says.

Instead of taking her scheduled lunch hour, Jane telephones the admitting office for the records of her afternoon appointments, orders a lithium-level determination for a patient, buys a bag of nuts at the vending machine, and rushes to the ampitheater of the center for the afternoon lecture. The speaker is a young visiting gynecologist who discusses contraceptive failure, explaining its frequency in various methods of birth control, some of the reasons, and the need for very concrete instructions to patients.

The audience consists of physicians, RNs, PAs, LPNs (licensed practical nurses), and aides, many of whom sit munching their brown-bag lunches. The noontime lecture-discussion is a feature of the center's in-service training, with several visiting authorities scheduled each week. Attendance is voluntary, but as a rule, at least forty persons attend, more or less on a selective basis. Many participate actively during the question-and-answer period.

Back in her own office, Jane telephones an allergy patient of one of the team doctors. (Even when no one answers a call, she makes a notation in the record of the day and hour.) A detailed conversation follows, Jane asking questions and making suggestions as to the presence of mold, wool, dust, pillows, and the use of air conditioning and antihistamines, as well as the pros and cons of allergy testing and desensitization injections. The decision whether to undergo the testing is to be made by the patient.

A new member of the health center, about forty years of age, arrives for his initial health check. He tells Jane that he "understands what a PA is all about," for his wife, a graduate of the Duke program, works in one of the drug-control outpatient clinics at the university medical center.

Like Geoffrey Francoeur, Jane is thorough, unhurried, and sensitive, both in the examination and the enormously important history taking. Laboratory tests are ordered, including one for white-corpuscle count.

Two urgent telephone calls await Jane. One of the center members has been in a motor accident and now finds himself in an out-of-state hospital. Since the center underwrites the cost of hospitalization wherever it may occur, Jane immediately contacts both the patient and the hospital.

The other message is from the pharmacy of the local general hospital. A patient of the center has presented herself in a bold ploy to procure a sleeping pill allegedly prescribed by Jane. Jane tells the pharmacy that she has given the patient no such prescription. But the call helps solve a mystery that has been plaguing the health-care center: a prescription pad is missing. Now it becomes obvious that this particular patient must have stolen it. Precautions are issued to the center's staff to keep stricter controls on all such pads.

A frail, charming lady of seventy-seven with a kidney and gallbladder problem . . . a woman whose Pap smear has disclosed the disease-causing organism Trichomonas . . . a young man with warts to be "frozen off" . . . a woman with a questionable mammogram who needs reassurance and help with next-step planning . . . records to keep current . . . numerous telephone calls from anxious patients . . .

This is Jane's day.

Jane, it goes without saying, is an intelligent, enthusiastic, extremely energetic young woman who is practicing medicine.

Quick, perceptive, knowledgeable, forever learning, she has much to offer her patients and the medical team of which she is part. She respects her limits and is honest about them. She has great conviction and integrity about her work. Her only source of unhappiness is that she is not being encouraged to go beyond it—to return to medical school and become a doctor.

The physicians with whom she works, perhaps selfishly, value Jane's contribution and are aware of her special strengths. She is, in her present role, an excellent interpreter of medical data. She takes a splendid medical history, noting each significant clue. Her telephone sessions with patients are never brusque, preoccupied grunts. Hers is a careful, purposive relationship, extending definite help, information, or support.

She is kept busy, very busy—she is called upon, during the busy day just described, to help the overloaded PA in another unit!—but she never conveys a sense of haste to the patient. Those concerned about the quality of medical care in our time should feel very encouraged that there are Geoffrey Francoeurs and Jane Dickinsons among us.

2

SOME BASIC QUESTIONS

What, exactly, is a PA?

A PA is a member of a complex profession based on a simple premise—that many medical tasks can be successfully performed by persons who are not full-fledged doctors. These may be *diagnostic* (finding out what is wrong) or *therapeutic* (deciding upon the treatment or cure).

The new health professionals are carefully trained in specific medical techniques. They may then practice these techniques under the supervision of a doctor.

Why haven't I known about PAs?

The field is still relatively young, and PAs are not yet numerous.

The idea was born at Duke University Medical

School in Durham, North Carolina, where the pilot
program was established in 1965–66. The next few years
saw the beginnings of similar programs at the Universities of Kansas and Colorado. Within five years after the
Duke groundwork was laid, fourteen PA programs had
been established.

In 1972 federal support, under the Bureau of
Health Manpower of the National Institutes of Health,
Education, and Welfare, gave additional impetus to the
movement. There are today forty-five accredited programs in twenty-eight states.

What kind of medical procedures may be done by PAs?
An impressive number.

1. The PA obtains thorough and detailed medical
histories from patients. This is a skill of immeasurable
importance in diagnosis.

2. The PA does comprehensive physical examinations of both children and adults.

3. The PA does routine technical tests (such as
gastric analysis, electrocardiograph, and pulmonary-
function testing) and explains the procedures and findings to patients.

4. The PA counsels patients concerning health care,
family planning, and therapy.

5. The PA monitors the condition of the sick.

6. The PA is skilled at suturing wounds and changing dressings.

7. The PA can apply and remove splints and casts.

8. The PA can perform routine screening, such as
Pap smear, tuberculin testing, and audiovisual mea-
surements.

9. The PA makes use of skills mastered in the course of training to meet the requirements of a specific practice. That practice may be a specialized one.

Are PAs then partially trained doctors?

Yes, but "partially trained" should by no means suggest "inadequately trained." They are thoroughly trained within a limited range of services.

Jeanne Fisher, director of admissions of the Johns Hopkins University School of Health Services, which trains PAs, believes graduates "are capable of delivering a major portion of the total services in a comprehensive health-care program."

She goes on to say, "We believe that students who graduate from this program will be well educated and professionally competent individuals who will have an important impact on the health-care delivery in the United States."

Most of our needs as patients do not require complex and sophisticated medical techniques. These remain, of course, the province of the physician, and when routine tasks are taken off his shoulders, he is free to concentrate on these more demanding cases. Moreover, since the education of the PA has been concentrated upon specific routine procedures, these are often performed less hurriedly, more earnestly, and perhaps more efficiently by a PA than a doctor. Many doctors are bored by run-of-the-mill cases (as a mathematician may be bored at the thought of adding up the household bills), whereas PAs may treat them with care and solicitude.

Within the next ten to twenty years, the PA may be

universally accepted as *the* medical person who does routine procedures best.

What's the difference between a physician's associate and a physician's assistant?
There are none. These terms are used interchangeably.

Also in use are the terms "health associate," "health practitioner," "primary-care physician's associate (or assistant)," and "medex," as well as "surgeon's assistant" and "urological physician's assistant." "Physician's assistant" is the most widely used.

Is there really a doctor shortage?
Definitely, although not everywhere. In a large city or in a medical center with a teaching hospital, there is usually no real shortage. But in large cities many urban poor have no family doctor and often use overcrowded hospital outpatient facilities for all their health problems. In small towns and rural areas, the shortage is even more pronounced. The PA programs were started—at least in part—to deal with such uneven distribution of health-care facilities.

Why don't they train more doctors instead of PAs?
Blunt economics. It has become astronomically expensive to educate a doctor.

Moreover, a great majority of American-trained physicians tend to specialize, which does not greatly increase the supply of primary-care physicians. Specialization tends to make educational costs—and patient fees—even higher.

Who were the first PAs, back in the midsixties?

It is a bizarre fact that PA beginnings are indebted to the Vietnam War, the most unpopular and disputed war in the memory of living Americans.

The emergency nature of war hastens the deployment of new medical and surgical techniques, new drugs, new methods of caring for the wounded. It is a time when taking a medical risk may prove more prudent than failure to do so, a time when necessity prompts experimentation.

The Army, Navy, and Air Force have a long history of training medical corpsmen for a variety of responsibilities and tasks. Long before general hospitals began to do so, the military refined their teaching procedures, gearing them to producing well-trained *technicians*. Each technician was taught to contribute a set of procedures essential to patient recuperation and wellbeing.

Not surprisingly, the earliest PAs were primarily ex-corpsmen, whose discipline and experience made them promising candidates for this new career. The Viet veteran with several years' service in a field hospital or a hospital ship seemed a natural. His preservice educational background was at first regarded as of secondary importance. It was his *experience* that mattered.

To this day experience remains a point of emphasis in spelling out admissions requirements for PA candidates. As the Vietnam War recedes in time, however, we find fewer ex-corpsmen among PA candidates and a greater importance attached to educational preparation, particularly in the sciences.

You mean someone like Geoffrey Francoeur couldn't make it today?

Educational requirements are now higher. Perhaps Geoffrey would find admission to the program he elected more difficult, but not altogether impossible. See pages 61-64 for further information on what to do if your educational background is inadequate for entry into a PA program.

Then why is experience still considered so important?

To begin with, experience has come to mean many things—almost any kind of work, volunteer and paid, in a health field involving direct contact with patients. It is not an absolute "must" in all schools, but such experience is valued by some of them as orientation to health careers and as a self-screening device. One learns very quickly, as aide or orderly, whether one will be content to spend one's working life, not necessarily as aide or orderly, but in the service of the ailing, the dying, the depressed, the diseased.

How can a high-school or college student get such experience?

Most hospitals have active volunteer offices. A willing volunteer, however young, is welcomed with open arms. Frequently there is a choice in the type of service one may select. Should this be the case, *direct patient care* of any sort should prove useful to future PAs.

Part-time paying jobs as nurse's aides and orderlies are available in hospitals and nursing homes. Weekend relief work provides an excellent entry. Full-time summer opportunities are sometimes available, although you must apply early for these.

Since a PA completes some of the education of a doctor, may he/she go on to medical school with advanced standing?

No. Although the PA does perform some of the functions of a doctor, his courses are not applicable, at this time, to a medical degree.

How do physicians feel about PAs?

Those doctors who have worked with PAs tend to be enthusiastic. Dr. Frank Woolsey, Jr., of the Albany–Hudson Valley Physician's Associate Program, quotes an internist in family practice who has employed a PA. "I feel less harried and I'm enjoying practice more. In a growing community, I couldn't take new patients. With the PA I can. . . . He sees all patients having certain complaints." (In other words, his PA handled that "major portion" of routine complaints mentioned earlier by Jeanne Fisher.)

A leading Connecticut orthopedist who used to scoff at the PA as "a superficially trained practical nurse with lots of theory," recently hired a young graduate for his office. This former skeptic was astonished and gratified by the results.

"My practice had reached the point where I either had to seek an associate—an M.D. completing his orthopedic residency—or take on a PA," he admits. "The former would have cut my income by a third at the very beginning, even more thereafter, and maybe louse up my estate when the time came. But this fellow is remarkable—he's worth his weight in gold, does some things better than I do. He's making it possible for me to extend my practice while actually spending more time with my family than I ever have. How about that?"

There have been pockets of resistance among individual doctors, but most of this breaks down as the word gets out about PAs and doctors cease to feel threatened by the newcomers. Only one state, New Jersey, has organized medical opposition to PAs.

How long must I study to become a PA?

One accredited program lasts only 12 months, but most require longer study than that—15, 16, 18, 23, 24, 27, and up to 42 months.

Moreover, some offer certificates upon completion, some an Associate in Science or Associate in Arts degree; others award a Bachelor of Science or Bachelor of Arts. A few may lead to the Master's degree.

Most PA programs are taught in medical schools, which in turn are part of larger universities. Others are connected with institutions that have no medical schools, although allied health careers may be taught.

Two are directly administered by the military. These, which should not be confused with courses for corpsmen, are AMA approved schools for the training of PAs. One is sponsored by the Medical Center for Federal Prisoners. Others are part of community colleges.

Then there must be different kinds of physicians' associates?

Of course. Assistants to physicians are divided into three general types.

Type A: Physician's associate, with duties described earlier in Chapter 2. Education frequently involves two entire years. The PA may assist either a primary-care physician or a specialist, having been trained in a variety of skills. A statement issued by George Washington University's School of Medicine and Health Sciences says of its trainees: "The assistant must possess enough knowledge of medicine to permit some degree of independent action within defined rules and circumstances and to perform properly at this level."

Type B: The title is the same, but the training is narrower and applicable only to a particular specialty. For example, there is a Surgeon's Assistant Program and a Urologic Physician's Program. According to the same George Washington University source, a student thus trained "is, as a result, less capable of independent action, but within his area of skill and knowledge, he may be equal to the Type A assistant *or the physician himself.* . . ."

Type C: An aide who is taught, either informally or by an employer or in a short-term vocational course, to perform one or more tasks for a physician, a group practice, or a hospital. No decision making or independent judgment is required. Such programs are not accredited and are outside the scope of this book.

The majority of schools approved by the American Medical Association (AMA), irrespective of their admissions requirements or the level of their degree, offer Type A education.

3

CHOOSING A PA CAREER

Ralph and Ellen were high-school steadies. One of the things that brought them together was their interest in health care. Ellen wanted to be a nurse, Ralph a doctor. Or they thought they did. But young people's plans have a way of going awry, and that's what happened here.

Ellen's Story

Ellen was a bright girl. She had always enjoyed school, and it was understood that she'd be class salutatorian at the end of term. But as she met her boyfriend after school one day, she was unhappy.

"Hey, what's the matter?" Ralph asked.

"It's my counselor. She thinks I should do a volunteer stint at the V.A. hospital. It'll burn up two afternoons a week."

"What brought that on? She never told *me* to do that."

"Well, It's because I'm applying to nursing. She said it's one way of being sure that's what I want. In a health career, she says, it's yes or no, never in between."

"Sounds reasonable. Why not try it?"

"I suppose I'll have to."

Ellen joined a group of high-school students doing volunteer work two or three afternoons a week. She was surprised to learn that the V.A. hospital employed a full-time professional to recruit and orient volunteers. Some of her classmates chose to work in administrative service, X-ray department, admissions, physical therapy, or in one of the many outpatient clinics. With her counselor's words in mind, Ellen chose nursing service and was assigned to a surgical ward.

It did not take more than a few weeks for Ellen to realize the wisdom of the experiment. She first discussed the problem with Ralph. "I knew I'd find unpleasant things in a hospital—pain and suffering, sights, smells, bedpans—you know," she said. "I was prepared for all that. But what upset me—what *really* upset me was—people."

"Come again? You lost me somewhere."

"Well, you walk into a ward or somebody's room. Everybody looks up. And you've got to—you know—smile and say something nice and cheerful. You've got to *talk* to them, all the while you're doing what you're there

to do. Be clever or funny. Ooze what they call empathy. I think it's the people I can't take." And the tears
flowed.

"I don't understand you," said Ralph. "Of course
you're dealing with people. All the patients are *people*.
They're people before they're patients."

"I know. But that's what I find so hard. Like making
small talk on a bus all the way to—to California. . . ."

Ralph was confused, "But, Ellen, why did you go in
for nursing in the first place?"

I always thought I'd like it because I like science. But nursing isn't all science. It isn't even *mostly*
science. It's mostly people — and that's the part I can't
take!"

After a moment's thought, Ralph said, "I guess
you'd better find some other career in health care that
doesn't involve constant contact with patients.

And Ellen did. After several sessions with her
counselor, she decided to apply to the School of Allied
Health of the university instead of the School of Nursing.
There she majored in medical technology and did very
nicely among her test tubes.

Every young person who plans a career in the
health field, of whatever kind, should test himself with
volunteer work at a local hospital or clinic. Even a
negative experience like Ellen's is useful in determining
which branch of medicine to apply for, and of course
positive experiences occur, too. The volunteer may
discover a whole new kind of health-care career, which
he'd never thought of before but which exactly suits his
talents.

Ralph's Story

Unlike Ellen, Ralph had never been a scholar in high school. His grades ranged from average to good, and he had to work hard to get them.

Like many working-class families, Ralph's people held physicians in awe, so in college Ralph embarked on a premedical program. By the end of his second year, he had completed courses in general and organic chemistry, physics, zoology, biochemistry, mathematics, Spanish, English, art appreciation, sociology, and psychology. He did fairly well in them, but he had to work so hard that he came down with mononucleosis and lost his campus job, which he needed for financing his studies. And just then his father died. He found himself totally without funds.

Ralph decided to drop out of college for a year "to put my head together." He procured a job as orderly in a large city hospital. He was impressed by the interns, residents, and medical students, but discouraged by the thought of the long years of study and the huge financial outlay that would be needed to pursue a career in medicine.

At the hospital he met and was befriended by several young men and women from a nearby PA program. They were performing their "clerkships," a series of experience blocks similar to a rotating internship. Up to that time Ralph had never heard of a PA.

He shared his excitement with his mother and with Ellen. Practical, methodical Ellen suggested he pay a visit to his former premedical adviser, a professor of biochemistry at the university. Ralph made the appointment with some qualms, wondering whether Dr. Otto would consider the PA program a copout.

He was pleasantly surprised. Dr. Otto proved enthusiastic and extremely knowledgeable. He advised Ralph where to send for information, appraised several educational programs with which he had some personal contact, and said (in answer to Ralph's halting query) that, yes, he would gladly write a reference letter for him.

Professor Otto also gave Ralph a mimeographed sheet which, he said, he used as a little test for some of his students who aspired to a health career.

At Ralph's startled look, Dr. Otto laughed. "You won't get graded on it, so just sit back and work quickly and comfortably. Each question calls for an answer of yes or no. Don't hesitate or ponder. Give the answer that immediately occurs to you—I want your gut reaction."

1. Am I compassionate? Am I deeply concerned about people and their well-being?

2. Am I committed to helping, whether I like or dislike the recipients, whether I think them worthy or unworthy, to the best of my ability, knowledge, and skills?

3. Am I relatively mature? Am I emotionally stable? (Be rough on yourself.)

4. Can I graciously accept irregular and unpopular hours, evening, weekend, and holiday responsibilities, and sometimes a sense of injustice about the apportionment of such responsibilities?

5. Am I intellectually adequate to the challenge of this career? Am I a questing person? Do I

really want to *know*, or do I regard education merely as a union card to a good job?

6. Have I acquired fastidious study skills and can I stick with an assignment or a task until it is finished, even though I may be exhausted?

7. Have I learned to take pains with everything I do, even an application blank?

8. Do I have excellent health and real stamina? Can I work under extreme pressure?

9. Am I intelligent? Have I already proved my ability to handle difficult subject matter?

10. Would I feel pride and a sense of personal achievement if admitted to this profession?

Ralph put his pen away and looked up. "They're all yeses."

"All? Every single one of them?"

"Every one of them."

"Even your weekend covering emergencies while the doctor is out on the golf course getting a nice tan?"

"Even."

"What about the rapist-murderer-thug brought in with a bullet in his stomach—what's so terrible, Ralph, if he dies?"

"That's the court's problem," said Ralph. "My job isn't to like him—my job is to see that he lives."

"You have worked all night and it's seven A.M. Your relief doesn't show. What then?"

"I'd take two cups of black coffee and wash my face in cold water."

Professor Otto laughed and shook hands with Ralph. "I think you're going to be a good PA," he predicted.

What PAs Must Expect to Be

As Professor Otto's list of questions pointed up, the PA's job is, above all, people oriented. The PA must be someone who is deeply concerned about the health and well-being of others and basically motivated by this concern.

You may protest that you know doctors, very capable and successful ones, who do not seem at all people-oriented. Indeed, many are shy and withdrawn persons or quick, sarcastic smart alecks, who are highly successful at concealing any lurking compassion they may feel for sick people.

It's true that there are such physicians among us. Many men and women are drawn into medicine because of their interest in disease or physiological function, which they manage to dissociate entirely from the human beings who contain them. They may remain aloof or disagreeable toward patients at all times and are tolerated only because they are extraordinarily good at their jobs.

The PA, however, is the person the doctor would entrust with the delicate business of patient relationships. This means the explaining and discussing, the calming and encouraging, the answering of questions—wise, foolish, repetitive—the numerous details of a doctor-patient relationship that the physician does not always have the time or the temperament to nurture. The PA can convey to patients that person-to-person element which medicine seems to have lost, except among the white-coated heroes of the TV screen.

People-oriented does not necessarily mean popular or even socially gregarious. Popularity or lack of it is less

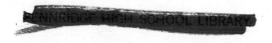

important than whether one is concerned, sympathetic, anxious to be of help to others. And as Ralph told the professor, the PA's job is not to like the patient but to cure him, because—saint or criminal—he is a human being.

With that one reply, Ralph proved himself both people-oriented and nonjudgmental. Later on—the professor shrewdly guessed—Ralph would not be ill-tempered with a fifteen-year-old patient because he contracted syphilis or she had gotten pregnant out of wedlock. He would make no grandstand speeches to the middle-aged alcoholic or the overweight housewife. His sole concern would be to snuff out an ugly health problem and to see his patient protected against a recurrence.

The PA must willingly devote himself to his profession. Do you require regular working hours? Are your weekends sacrosanct and your holidays inviolable? Would you be wretched if obliged to work rotating hours—usually 7:00 A.M. to 3:00 P.M., 3:00 P.M. to 11:00 P.M., and 11:00 P.M. to 7:00 A.M., each shift lasting a week or more? Would you sulk if you had to work on Christmas Day or Thanksgiving, when all your friends are home from college or when your entire family is together?

Conditions of employment in health careers must be geared to the needs of the sick. And the sick, alas, do not suspend their illness because it is Saturday or Sunday, New Year's Eve or the Fourth of July. We have all seen ambulances tearing down big city streets at night, sirens howling, rushing to disgorge disaster victims or the suddenly stricken at a hospital. There has

to be hospital personnel to receive them, whether it is five in the morning or midnight of a legal holiday.

This must be borne in mind when deciding upon a health career. Hours may be more or less regular for a PA, but there will be the odd shift, the rotating one, some or other emergency, particularly at the beginning of one's career. Friday night's problem will not keep till Monday.

Television has helped make health careers glamorous, perhaps somewhat unreal. Many young persons, excited by such programs, begin to see themselves in a white coat, face mask, and rubber gloves, engaging in a melodramatic career that, whatever its setbacks, is ultimately crowned with success. All lives will be saved, all problems ironed out, all operations acts of triumphant wizardry.

Actually, the PA, like other health professionals, is a very hard worker, often exhausted and bone-weary, sometimes eating and sleeping irregularly, sometimes troubled by baffling problems for which there are no solutions. Nevertheless, although the family doctor no longer makes house calls or wears his dedication on his sleeve, dedication is demanded from the PA, who is still working for total acceptance.

Indeed, the PA will often be the one person on the medical team from whom old-fashioned GP qualities will be taken for granted. The physician may be gruff, uncommunicative, busy; his crowded office will tell you why and his patients accept it. The PA will be expected to do an *unhurried* examination and satisfy the most anxious or unpleasant patients. That is why he or she is there.

The PA must also be intelligent. Warmth, empathy, ease of relating, belief in the worth and dignity of the least among us—these are important, but they are not enough.

A PA, like other health professionals, has a huge amount to learn and absorb and retain during the typical twenty-four-month educational program. For the person who tends to be slow, superficial, content with an average performance, or lacking in diligence, such a program would prove staggering.

In other words, this is a career for the hard-working, above-average student who has already demonstrated an ability to handle difficult subjects, who is disciplined, memorizes without agony, and can study, understand, and assimilate learning under conditions of fatigue and stress.

4

APPLYING TO
PA PROGRAMS

Application

Admissions officers are frequently exasperated by the condition of applications sent in by would-be students. If yours is careless, smudged, streaked, dog-eared, crossed-out, ungrammatical, or incompletely assembled, the admissions board will identify you as sloppy, too, and you will soon find yourself reading one of those "Due to a large volume of qualified applicants, we regret to advise . . ." replies. This does *not* mean that you will be graded on neatness and penmanship alone. It means that this application is worth taking pains over—this one and all the others. It will be read and carefully considered, but don't make handicaps for yourself.

The application indicates to the admissions board whether or not you are technically eligible for their program in PA education. But it does much more than that. It introduces you to them, with hints of your thoroughness, the efforts you are willing to invest in your education, your dedication and competence for a career that demands exactitude.

So, take pains with the application blank. Fill out answers to the questions on a practice sheet first. Then if you change your mind on one point or find that you have misread a question, you can cross out and correct to your heart's content. When you have every answer just the way you want it, then copy the information onto the application blank proper—neatly and legibly.

The *applicant's statement* (a blank page offering an opportunity to say exactly what the candidate wants to tell the admissions committee) should be taken seriously. Some programs ask a motivation question—why you want to become a PA or where you became acquainted with the career or the program. Write out a rough pencil draft first; reread, correct, and refine it as you did with the application blank, before you send it off in its final form.

Applying to a professional program in the health field is a process requiring one's best efforts and a generous allocation of time and attention. If you need to lock yourself into your room for a weekend—or several weekends—it is worth the time, for it is worth doing well.

Since places are limited, each candidate should make his or her application as interesting, readable, and accurate as possible. A hearts-and-flowers approach—

downright sentimentality about how you bleed over the poor unfortunates of the world—should be avoided. Dedication *is* part of the package, but it should be possible to indicate the proper attitude without dissolving into self-congratulation.

Allow yourself sufficient time to get everything you will need. Many applications are sent by students who have already completed some college work. This frequently means that two sets of records, high school and college, must be sent for, as well as proof of work experience, SAT scores, and recommendations—a time-consuming process. Whatever your circumstances may be, it makes sense to start the application procedure early and plan it with care.

Letters of Reference

How important are references—really? Young people are often casual, if not actually flippant, about their letters of recommendation.

The following guidelines should be observed in seeking or designating references for your application.

1. Before you put down someone's name as a possible reference, ask permission of that person. He may not want the bother of writing a recommendation at all, or—embarrassing situation—he may not feel that you merit it. Give him the courtesy of choice.

2. To write a meaningful reference, one must know the candidate well enough to be able to judge how appropriate the application is. Don't corral someone who knows you only slightly.

3. Remember that teachers, counselors, family doctors, and former employers do not routinely write glowing recommendations. Don't expect a Niagara of unwarranted praise.

4. If the person you are approaching for the reference seems reluctant, accept this graciously as a refusal and do not force the issue. His reasons may have nothing to do with you. He may be swamped with other paperwork; he may have a temperamental distaste for writing recommendations; he may be a slow, cumbersome writer. Withdraw your request and continue the hunt.

5. Seek out *logical* references. Those in a position to judge your performance in a health setting are particularly serviceable. Your scholastic ability, motivation, past performance, industry, and study skills are factors your references may be asked to evaluate. Of real use are recommendations from those who have been your science instructors and those who have taught and graded you in English and communication skills.

6. A valid reference is always *confidential* between the writer and the admissions board, and it must be mailed *by the writer*. However, it is thoughtful and courteous of you to submit with your request a neatly typed, stamped, and correctly addressed envelope, which bears the return address of the person who is giving the reference—*not yours*.

Never ask a person to hand over a letter of reference for you to post, even on the pretext that it will accompany other materials or that your instructions require this (they won't). A reference mailed by you is of no value and will be discounted by the admissions board.

7. Give the writer time to compose a fair and carefully-thought-through recommendation. If there is a deadline, that is *your* headache. Make the request early enough that the writer has ample leisure to fit the writing of it into his busy schedule.

8. If you are uneasy and in doubt as to whether a promised letter has been dispatched, it is quite all right to ask, but do so *after a decent interval*. It is arrogant to expect a busy professional to drop everything and give your letter top priority, so wait two weeks to a month before asking. And ask tactfully.

Much of the above is simple application etiquette. Observing these suggestions will be appreciated by those writing on your behalf, and may result in warmer, more effective letters to support your candidacy.

These do's and don'ts are in no way intended to discourage what admissions people call the unusual applicant—the one whose preparation has been atypical, who is a product of an urban ghetto or a disadvantaged background, or who is older than the average candidate. All colleges and professional schools are interested in the unusual person. Many have made generous provisions to include minority students or those irregularly prepared. However, no PA program can accommodate a *totally unprepared* student or teach what should have been learned years before.

Making up Educational Shortcomings

Some higher education programs probably do open their doors to ill-prepared candidates, usually in an attempt to achieve racial, geographical, ethnic, or sex balance in their student bodies. But health programs cannot afford to lower their standards. The difference between good preparation and poor preparation may prove the difference between health and disease, life and death. In health education, there is too much at stake. Students must meet certain minimum requirements in order to be accepted.

How does one go about repairing poor preparation? With time, dedication, and much hard work.

A good first resource is the familiar territory of the high school. Many schools permit a limited number of recent graduates to attend a cost-free postgraduate year. This should be spent accumulating or beefing up basics: English, mathematics, laboratory sciences, all selected from among the most *demanding* courses offered.

The math, of course, must begin at the level where you left off. However, since some forms of math— algebra and geometry, for example—are unrelated (that is, you can understand either without having studied the other), it is possible to carry courses in both at the same time. But that's not an easy assignment.

High-school and college counselors are aware of requirements for health-care programs. Their experience with candidates, successful and unsuccessful, has given them a sensitivity that goes beyond a mere spelling out of those requirements. Listen to what they advise.

There are numerous private organizations that engage in vocational testing and counseling. B'nai Brith does this competently on a national and nonsectarian basis. Many universities open such services to persons outside the student community. Although a fee is normally charged by these private agencies, it is usually based on the individual's ability to pay.

The continuing-education programs of nearby colleges, YMCAs and YWCAs, community centers, and public night schools may offer helpful courses in communication skills, mathematical concepts, and the sciences. These are worth exploring.

Careful inquiries to local colleges, public and private, may disclose summer programs, some funded by the federal government, for the purpose of helping the disadvantaged applicant prepare for a health career. Sometimes a day spent at the telephone will yield excellent prospects. Some of these programs actually pay the student a stipend while strengthening his or her qualifications. However, these grants are a year-to-year enterprise; an accurate listing is impossible. Interested persons might direct an inquiry to the *Department of Health, Education, and Welfare, Health Resources Administration, 9000 Rockville Pike, Bethesda, Maryland 20014*, requesting a list of recent or ongoing projects. Once this is available, it is best to communicate directly with the college that offers such programs.

Perhaps the most promising resources of all lie in the community colleges that have mushroomed in every state in the union. Today few Americans have no community college within comfortable commuting distance of their homes. Most CCs have an open admissions policy, meaning that everyone may be admitted for a general education. Tuition costs are very low (some schools charge no tuition); many schedule classes in the late afternoon or evening; all are geared to work with the student whose preparation is deficient or weak. Moreover, community colleges are friendly and hospitable to the *older* student.

A year spent in a solid liberal-arts program at a community college should greatly strengthen an applicant's credentials. Two years in a community college, with a logical choice of subjects, would qualify many for degree-granting health programs. Added to a secondary school record, however shallow, such an experience can prove rewarding. It tells admission staffs that the candidate has become aware of his existing shortcomings and is in the process of correcting them—that this applicant has learned academic discipline.

A student who has avoided difficult subjects, then, throughout high school, can enter a community college, speak frankly with a counselor concerning his or her long-range goals, and begin a sequence of appropriate subjects in a friendly, noncompetitive environment. Community colleges are frequently a last chance for those who missed their high-school opportunities.

5

THE EDUCATION OF A PA

To his great relief and satisfaction, Ralph was accepted by the school to which he applied. He presented himself eagerly in early September and was handed a list of courses and classroom hours to be completed. For an uneasy instant, he thought he was the victim of a practical joke:

Anatomy (lecture and laboratory)	145 hours
Animal surgery	46 hours
Bacteriology	22 hours
Basic clinical laboratory (hematology, urinalysis, chemistries)	46 hours
Electrocardiography and cardiac care	22 hours
Emergency treatment and management	48 hours
Epidemiology and public health	16 hours

Ethical and legal aspects of medicine	8 hours
Family practice seminar	22 hours
History taking and physical examination	80 hours
Human development (embryology)	54 hours
Human sexuality	22 hours
Integrated physiology and biochemistry	90 hours
Interviewing techniques	30 hours
Introduction to clinical medicine and surgery	272 hours
Pathology	24 hours
Pharmacology	60 hours
Psychodynamics of human behavior	60 hours
Radiology	24 hours
Social medicine	18 hours

These courses were to be followed by a series of five-week blocks of clinical experiences or "clerkships," comparable to the medical student's rotating internship, with endless round-the-clock hours and responsibilities. Ralph would have to complete twelve of these—seven of them required of all candidates and five electives chosen by him.

His required clerkships would be these: emergency services, family practice, general surgery, internal medicine, obstetrics and gynecology, pediatrics, and psychiatry. The choice of electives was broad enough to give Ralph a direction for his future practice. They were cardiology, chemotherapy-oncology (oncology is the study of tumors), continuing care, dermatology, medical outpatient clinic, neurology, neurosurgery, orthopedic surgery, otolaryngology (the study of the ear, nose, and throat), pediatric surgery, trauma, and urology.

All courses had to be passed, of course; a single failure would eliminate Ralph from the program.

Apart from the five electives, there is no choice as to what one will and will not study. PA programs allow no such thing as "creating one's own curriculum"—no shopping around for a sympathetic professor, no opportunities for "trying out." The body of medical knowledge to be mastered is so vast that only a prescribed, structured course of study will produce employable graduates.

Such a pattern prevails in virtually all programs, Ralph learned. Credit for previous work is never granted. (Previous work may be recognized toward a degree or prove helpful in gaining admission, but the actual number of hours spent in a PA program may not be reduced by virtue of prior work in any other program.) There may be differences between programs in the length of training or in focus (whether general or specialized) or in the names given particular courses. But even where no degree is offered, the career program is prescribed and must be mastered *without exception*.

From the Ground up

It began for Ralph, as it begins for most future doctors, with a course in gross human anatomy, which met every morning of the week for a concentrated three hours.

"Not similar to—the same course!" he told Ellen excitedly. Facing his first cadaver and making his first incision with a somewhat unsteady scalpel had been as

dramatic—and trying—a moment as it is for most
first-year medical students. For a few minutes, Ralph
had felt very, very queasy.

"They can't expect the same from you as from those
medical students," Ellen protested.

"They sure do."

"I don't get it. If you're taking the same courses as
the medical students, why aren't you considered a
medical student, too? What's the difference?"

"You have to think of it as four years versus two
years. I'm getting medical training, all right, but a lot
less of it. I'll be a PA in two years. The med student
needs four for his MD, plus an internship, and if he
specializes, he'll be around cramming another two to six
years. So ultimately he will know a *lot* more than I do,
though for the moment we sit side by side in certain
classes."

In the animal surgery course Ralph quickly learned
sterile techniques, how to administer anesthetics, the
use of respirators, and basic surgical procedures. Because he loved animals, he approached each problem
with concern and a supreme effort to do his very best.
When one of his dog patients died, Ralph felt sadness,
but the death taught him an unforgettable lesson about
cardiac arrest.

Because he entered the program with a strong
background in the sciences, Ralph did not find the
clinical laboratory course difficult. He had always enjoyed chemistry and chemical experiments and was soon
able to do a complete blood work-up and a careful
urinalysis. These procedures were everyday tools in
diagnosis and treatment.

Ralph also became expert in electrocardiography, learning to handle the machinery quickly and competently. Above all, he enjoyed his evaluation sessions with prominent heart specialists, and spent many evenings in the medical-school library over recent books and articles to supplement his newfound interest in cardiopulmonary disease.

Ralph was pleased that his course in emergency medicine was taught by graduate PAs, in addition to the physician. The young men and women who taught this course brought in and shared their diversified clinical experiences in hospital emergency rooms and the offices of private practitioners. Ralph learned about medical, psychiatric, and obstetrical emergencies, how to identify them, how to handle them. Such trauma as head and neck injuries, multiple fractures, massive bleeding, shock, airway obstruction, pulmonary edema, allergic reactions, diabetic crises, endocrine emergencies, convulsion, burns, hand injuries, psychotic and suicidal episodes, drug and narcotic overdose, septic abortion, obstetrical bleeding, and common children's emergencies were part of this course.

A special interest in psychiatric emergencies again drove Ralph to the medical-school library. He was delighted that, as a PA in training, he was permitted to participate in the psychopathology course of the medical school, learning by lecture, one-way screen, and videotape to recognize and understand neuroses, psychoses, and organic brain illness.

History taking, a skill of great importance in making a diagnosis, was combined with methods of performing a complete physical examination. The ability to interview

patients carefully and pointedly was stressed, with audio
and videotaped sessions used for class analysis. Ralph
then had opportunities to interview clinic patients under
very close supervision, and to discuss the histories and
diagnostic clues with his professors.

As preparation for his future studies in clinical
medicine, Ralph completed a course in human development, normal and abnormal, involving a review of
biology from simplest to most complex forms of life.
Again he was grateful for his strong science background.
"I wouldn't have survived without it," he admitted to
Ellen. "The time pressure alone would have made me a
casualty. As it is, I keep running all the time. I never
before realized how much you can squeeze into twenty-
four hours. . . ."

Most rewarding to Ralph during the first nine
months of the program was the all-important introduc-
tory course in clinical medicine and surgery. This was
regarded as an interdisciplinary course—that is, it drew
upon the knowledge and experience of many kinds of
professionals. To his great amazement, lectures were
given by doctors, nurses, physical therapists, dietitians,
PAs, and other members of the health team. Audiovisual
aids, such as movies, slides, specimens, models, and X
rays were used in the presentations.

And at long last, Ralph began to make hospital
rounds—at first merely observing and asking questions,
in time becoming involved in the actual treatment of
patients.

It was the aim of the program to provide Ralph with
so varied an experience that he would be able to work in
any setting and undertake competently any task, no

matter what degree of skill and responsibility it would demand.

Ralph was assigned specific patients admitted to the university hospital, both in the wards and in the private pavilion. Sometimes a patient was admitted from the emergency room. One of his early patients thus admitted was a tiny, elderly woman, unconscious after a massive stroke. Ralph checked for vital signs, conferred with internist and neurologist concerning his diagnosis and the extent of the stroke, ordered and set up intravenous apparatus and the machinery required for nourishment.

Working swiftly and purposively under the watchful eyes of experienced doctors, Ralph felt a surge of exhilaration. All at once he knew what had caused him to seek a career in the health field.

"I'm fighting for a life," he realized. "I'm literally fighting for a life. . . ."

Later, as his patient improved, Ralph watched her daily progress, conferred again with both physicians and physical therapist, and spent several hours interpreting the findings to members of the patient's family. It was a happy day for him when he discharged her to a nursing home, where she would complete her recovery.

In the pediatric ward, Ralph was assigned to a child with leukemia—a tense, frightened eleven-year-old who had to be introduced to the terror of chemotherapy. Ralph was gentle and patient, talked to the little girl about her friends and her pets, and offered to teach her to play chess, since she had already won all her checker games. Within a short time the child was calm and even cheerful about her coming ordeal, and Ralph had a new

friend. He was somewhat embarrassed when the little
girl told the specialist who had been called in that she
preferred to be treated by "Dr. Ralph."

Ralph worked with derelict alcoholics who had been
brought in by police ambulance. He also treated wealthy
private patients in the carpeted, air-conditioned pavilion, gaining experience in many specialties. He knew he
would be ready, when the time came, to work in any
setting. From the first he recognized that, whereas some
doctors would not entrust a PA with any procedure
("Masterson grabbed the hypodermic needle right out of
my hand!"), there were others who turned over virtually
all procedures to him, contenting themselves with a nod
and a mutter.

It would be like that when he completed his
education and entered the world of work. But he would
be prepared!

6

COSTS, REWARDS, AND THE JOB OUTLOOK FOR PAs

Ralph, by virtue of his own savings, a small insurance policy left him by his father, and a government-underwritten loan, managed to scrape together enough tuition money to carry him through his two years of training. Other would-be PAs might find it easier—or a lot harder.

Educational Costs

Suppose you had decided to apply to one of the new PA programs a decade ago. A pleasant surprise would have awaited you. In those days most of the programs were tuition-free.

Geoffrey and Jane paid no tuition fees and were

compelled to meet only the cost of food, shelter, and personal needs. Ralph, on the other hand, will pay $2,700 for his first year's tuition and several hundred dollars in fees. Luckily, he will continue to live at home; many students must pay room and board as well as tuition. Ralph anticipates that tuition costs may be even higher for the second year.

Today only a few MEDEX programs, those restricted to members of the armed services, and a government-sponsored one for the purpose of supplying health personnel to the Bureau of Prisons are available without payment of tuition and fees. A small number make token charges, mostly to state residents.

No longer experimental, most PA programs do exact tuition and a variety of miscellaneous fees. Costs vary from the nominal to the eyebrow raisers, with the highest charges being paid by students of private colleges and by out-of-state residents at public institutions.

Appendices 1 and 2 of this book offer sketches of each recognized program and indicate the costs that prevailed during the 1977–78 academic year.

In terms of costs, the future of education in the United States, particularly career education, will become more and more expensive. This trend reflects not only the increased costs of providing that education but supply and demand as well. More and more persons are seeking health careers each year.

How, then, should you plan the financing of a PA program?

First, you should sit down with the most recent estimate of expenses published by the college you plan to enter and work out a realistic and accurate budget. Start by listing the estimated cost of every item involved in your lifestyle: food, clothing, housing, cigarettes, telephone and long-distance calls, automobile and/or other travel expenses, stamps, stationery, toiletries, haircuts, bowling fees, stereo equipment, tennis fees, concert and movie admissions, etc.—in addition, of course, to the cost of books and school fees not included in tuition. It is wise to assume that your actual expenses will exceed your estimate by at least 10 percent and that the second year's expenses will exceed those of the first year by the same amount.

The total sum should be matched against your resources—all you have saved from jobs or military experience and all your family is willing or able to invest in your future. If resources fall short of expenses—as they often do—there are several ways to make up the difference.

Grants and Loans

1. The G.I. Bill, with its educational benefits, underwent many changes during the years following World War II. Early in 1977, it was allowed to expire. Persons who enlisted prior to its expiration will continue to draw benefits for a long time in the future, but persons who enlist in the service after that date must look for other forms of assistance.

The military services, however, have not retreated from their earlier commitment to education. Men and women enlistees receive tuition assistance totaling 75 percent of the cost of all educational courses in which they are enrolled while on active duty. Those who look forward to continuing education upon separation from the services may save up to $75 a month from their salaries for this purpose, with Uncle Sam contributing $2 to match each dollar saved by the enlistee. These savings must be specifically earmarked for education.

2. Where need is demonstrable, the Basic Educational Opportunity Grant (BEOG) may prove helpful. This consists of outright federal grants, which need not be repaid. The BEOG may provide up to $1,400 in a given year, although most grants are smaller. Information and applications are available at secondary and post-secondary schools and public libraries, or you may write directly to P.O. Box 84, Washington, D.C. 20044. Unfortunately, BEOG materials are made available rather late in the planning year, so that it becomes difficult to count on a grant well ahead of time. To compensate for the bureaucratic delay in issuing materials, applications are processed very quickly, usually within a month.

3. Another federal program, Supplementary Educational Opportunity Grant (SEOG), may provide an additional grant-in-aid for students with unusual financial need. Both this program and BEOG are for undergraduate work only. In both, eligibility is determined *by need alone*.

4. The Guaranteed Student Loan Program makes it possible for students to borrow directly from a local bank, because the loan is guaranteed by the state and insured by the federal government. These loans may be used to finance either graduate or undergraduate study.

Interest rates and loan ceilings differ from state to state. Ask your local savings bank to explain prevailing conditions and limitations. Since job prospects for the future PA appear to be excellent, it should not be too difficult to borrow on these expectations.

5. Partial scholarships and loans are available from regular college and university sources. The financial-aid office of the institution you wish to enter should be the *first* resource you approach for information and assistance in financing your education. This is true for both graduate and undergraduate education.

Work

1. Some programs offer students opportunities for part-time employment, preferring students with prior health-care experience. Others (and these are more numerous) discourage students from undertaking work while committed to so demanding a program as PA study. Free time is extremely limited during term, and vacation periods are brief, so unless your work is highly specialized, requiring little time and offering large pay, off-campus employment is not a good idea. However, financial-aid offices should prove helpful in finding jobs for the spouses (either sex) of enrolled PA students.

2. Preceptorships (blocks of experience as assistant in a doctor's office, part of the training in some programs) frequently offer a stipend, usually $250 to $350 per month. Not all programs, of course, have a preceptorship period.

Job Outlook and Rewards

After you have undergone this demanding and expensive education—invested your parents' savings or committed yourself to repay a substantial loan—what returns can you expect? Are there jobs waiting for the trained PA?

The answer is an emphatic yes. The job outlook today is excellent in all fields of health care. Here are some of the reasons why:

1. Heightened life expectancy. The number of senior citizens is increasing proportionally among our population, and the aged are large consumers of medical care.

2. Improved diagnostic and therapeutic techniques. These have actually created a new technology and the need for many new kinds of health workers.

3. Higher national standards of health maintenance.

4. Research wars against common killers such as cancer, heart disease, stroke, birth defects, and respiratory problems.

5. Numerous "detective projects" concerned with the environment. Whole teams of people are needed to study such factors as smog, water pollution, food additives and coloring, industrial waste, and other factors of modern living, to determine their effect on our lives.

We are now engaged in developing many specialists to cope with new conditions. Changes in health care point up the need for a steady supply of health personnel in the future. This is confirmed by the *Occupational Outlook Handbook*, 1976–77 edition, issued by the U.S. Department of Labor.

The greatest need in all of health care is for trained technicians to help physicians meet the enormous responsibilities of the future.

Looking ahead, the School of Allied Health Professions of the State University of New York at Stony Brook predicts that "openings for graduates of this program can be expected to increase markedly as the use and acceptance of PAs increases. Many physicians are already employing graduates, and it is evident that many more desire to hire accomplished graduates at the earliest possible date."

And Robert C. Creaser, chairman of the Department of Health Care Sciences of the University of Texas Medical Branch at Galveston says: "We believe that the role of the physician's associate offers a challenging and rewarding career, with an unlimited future for those who are willing to accept the responsibilities of the position."

Even those PAs who have encountered hostility from some individual physicians do not believe this has in any way limited their progress or made it difficult for them to obtain employment. On the contrary, most graduates have several offers to choose from in making a job decision. Three weeks after he came to his new position, Geoffrey Francoeur received a call from his former employer, representing the emergency room of a nearby general hospital. Would Geoffrey like to return? The welcome mat was out and his higher VA salary would be matched—topped, if need be.

Earnings

What does a PA earn? This is hard to state flatly in dollars and cents, because salaries vary from area to area, and inflation forces changes from one year to the next. However, the salary situation seems a healthy one for PAs. The first PA class of a large eastern university, few of whom had previous college-level education, found positions with starting salaries between $12,000 and $16,000.

Oddly, most practicing PAs seem to think their classmates are doing better than they financially. "I'm not in a position to set up shop in the backwater—where the real money is," explained one PA. "I've got two kids to educate." Another said, "Sure, if I wanted to take on an emergency-room graveyard shift, eleven to seven, including those beautiful Saturday nights when they come in on slabs after shootings, knifings, you name it—and the police are on your back before the job is done—sure, I could make more, but . . ."

But the choice was theirs to make.

Beginning PA salaries compare favorably with those of inexperienced college graduates in most fields. They are better than public schoolteachers' beginning salaries, on a level with engineers' perhaps, and better than those of most skilled health workers in other fields. It is too early to project the range or scope of possible advancement. By the middle 1980's, PAs will be more widely utilized in all fields of health care. In any case, the PA career, although difficult to enter, has much to offer the ambitious young man or woman.

As a rule, PAs employed by hospitals, private

physicians, and health-care centers work a standard forty-hour week. A few facilities continue to regard forty-four hours as standard, but these are the exception rather than the rule, and they are prepared to compensate the PA appropriately.

Still, the PA works long hours. There is the sheer volume of work to be gotten through, in addition to such tasks as keeping medical records current, conferring with physicians, answering the telephone, getting prescriptions countersigned, ordering and recording laboratory findings, absorbing in-service training, attending staff meetings, and so on.

Appointments are usually scheduled at precise times, but it is impossible to limit every patient to a prescribed fifteen, twenty, or thirty minutes. A thorough health check takes Jane Dickinson and Geoffrey Francoeur at least an hour, and a voluble or complex patient, especially one being seen for the first time, may well run this into an hour and a half. In the course of a busy day—most days are busy—this might well leave a backlog of patients still unseen at quitting time. But these patients cannot be dismissed simply because it is four thirty or five o'clock. So, a long day must often be made even longer.

In a hospital setting, PAs work closely with doctors, nurses, and an assortment of scientists, technologists, and technicians. To do this successfully, a PA must be tactful. Hospitals are very caste-conscious institutions. The PA's role is relatively new and not fully understood by the public or even all the health personnel. As an individual or a member of the team, the PA must be sensitive to the feelings and pretensions of others, guarded about his or her feelings, and absolutely devoid of pretensions of his own.

Despite all exigencies and crises, most modern city hospitals endeavor to keep standard working hours for the bulk of their employees, so you can count on a reasonable amount of leisure time. Three weeks to a month's vacation is usually part of the PA contract. Most health workers tend to take these free days in installments—that is, not at one time, but frequently clustered around legal holidays to lengthen the period and stretch out vacation possibilities. In this respect, PAs follow the pattern of salaried physicians and other hospital-based colleagues.

There is less certainty in rural practice. Isolated communities often lack a pool of medical personel to cover emergencies in rotation, and PAs provide an excellent way of filling the gap. Health-care centers, which are on the increase in many areas, need evening coverage for emergencies. Jane Dickinson works each Tuesday from twelve thirty until her last evening patient has been accommodated.

Still, as in most health careers, the results transcend dollars-and-cents considerations. The PA has the satisfaction of knowing his or her efforts may make the difference between living and dying, comfort and agony, health and disease. The material of the profession, human life, is very basic indeed. What the PA does is never unimportant or of dubious social value, and he knows that he is always needed.

7

HUMANIZING
MEDICAL CARE

Nowhere in a hospital does one see more panicky, desperate people than in the emergency room. Victims of accidents, crimes, fights . . . sudden heart attacks, fainting spells, seizures . . . patients who suddenly felt ill . . .

Colleen Lemaire, a PA in Emergency Service at Samaritan Hospital, has seen them all. "We get lots of serious emergencies—and lots of not-so-serious ones," she says. "Stretcher cases and cut fingers."

Colleen works from three in the afternoon until eleven at night, which she regards as the liveliest and most interesting shift for an emergency room. "The hospital itself is busiest during the morning and early afternoon, when most surgery and other forms of treatment are scheduled. But Emergency Service just starts picking up in the late afternoon. By evening things are hopping—and at night, wow!"

What will a typical evening bring?

"Well, yesterday we had two snow coronaries, one shooting victim, an alcoholic who'd fallen on his head and required seventeen stitches, an asthmatic baby, a young girl who'd been in an auto accident and needed an emergency tracheotomy (she couldn't breathe), and a middle-aged woman in shock. Dehydrated, no measurable pulse or blood pressure. All I could think of when they brought her in was terminal cancer. I wish I'd been wrong. . . ."

Do most patients arrive by ambulance?

"The very serious emergencies do. But most are brought in by families or friends. Some even walk in by themselves."

Colleen believes that Emergency Service has become the only source of medical help to many people, particularly those who live in cities—and not just the "urban poor."

"They don't have a family doctor, so they come to us. Or maybe they can't get a doctor because it's late at night or a weekend. Or their medical insurance won't cover a visit to a private physician but will cover an emergency visit to the hospital. Whatever the reason, we get them."

The hospital employs three PAs in Emergency Service, one during each shift. They work under the supervision of the director, a salaried M.D. who spends twelve hours a day, sometimes more, working along with his staff.

"I'd say Dr. Hitchcock is very happy with PAs in

Emergency," said Colleen. "We've speeded things up quite a bit, and we can be counted on to use good judgment. Even when we don't proceed on our own—I couldn't do a tracheotomy, of course—we know exactly what has to be done at once to relieve the patient and exactly whom to call. That can be very important."

She is quick to admit that economic factors play a part in the hospital's acceptance of the PA. At $14,500 each (starting salary) plus night differential (slightly higher rate for working the night shift), Colleen and her colleagues are delivering a lot of medical services at a relatively low cost. "And we're stable," she adds. "We live in this community, our families live here, whereas interns and residents keep changing all the time. Emergency Service may be just a stop along the way for them, but it's a career for us."

Colleen laughs. "I guess my bias is showing. Asking a PA to comment on PAs is like asking a chef whether the food is good. I think it's a terrific job, and I think we *do* a terrific job."

One of Colleen's teachers used to pound in an important lesson: "We're counting on you to humanize medicine."

"That's a tall order," says Colleen, "but we're doing it."

Patients Are People

Does medicine need humanizing? Many, including some doctors, believe that it does.

The physician, it is charged, has grown very aloof

from those he is pledged to serve. His time is immensely valuable. He finds it difficult or even irritating to communicate at any length with his patients. His competence, once he is licensed, is a matter of faith. If he makes an error in judgment or a medical sin of omission or commission, the patient's only recourse is an expensive and chancy lawsuit, which will chiefly enrich the lawyers involved. Since we need the doctor, we accept him at face value. But more and more we are beginning to dislike it.

In their dealings with patients, doctors are often gruff and unclear and make it plain that their time is precious, whereas ours is not. Most doctors no longer make house calls. They cover up for their own guild, even when there has been an obvious error or negligence. And they are expensive—often ludicrously so.

"When Medicare came in," an elderly woman tells Colleen Lemaire, "my doctor's charge for a visit went up double. From five dollars to ten. Even if he spent just two minutes with me and got called away to answer the phone, it was still ten dollars. It don't seem right. I mean, going up double on us older folks, all at once. When I asked him about it, reminded him I've been going to him twenty-two years, he told me I could go wherever I want."

She is shocked that modern medicine has grown impersonal and doctors less than enthusiastic about a patient who requires "reams" of Medicare paperwork. (Actually, it's only a one-page form.)

Many people denounce doctors as "money grubbers," and complain that their physicians are contemptuous and rude to them, often failing to warn them even about possible side effects of prescribed medication. And the poor feel strongly that they are not treated with dignity in the outpatient departments of some general hospitals.

"Everyone gets there at eight o'clock," grumbles an old man. "Then we wait an hour before an intern shows. If you're not fast when they call your name, you lose your turn. And sometimes they don't even tell you what the matter is. They just give you a slip for the druggist and tell you to come back next month."

Minority patients tell of doctors who convey an actual distaste for them. "He made me feel *nigger*," an educated black man reported of a well-known physician he had walked out on.

This last action was not an easy one to take. "He's got your history and a record of office visits, medication, all that," continued the indignant ex-patient. "He's already treating you. And you've paid him the seventy-five dollars for the first visit, the one with the tests, and a fortune since. It's pretty difficult and expensive to start all over again with another doctor."

But he felt so strongly about the specialist's attitude that he did do just that. The poor and the uneducated, however, have no choice but to submit to contempt.

Feminists claim that male physicians are callous toward women patients as *women*. Few obstetricians initially applauded the movement for natural, prepared childbirth. It was easier to keep contacts with the mother-to-be terse and routine throughout pregnancy and then to anesthetize her and deliver a drugged baby. "If men had the babies, they'd have made a more humane job of it long ago" is a common charge against the medical establishment.

Women doctors have remained relatively few in

number in the United States, a fact that continues to amaze Russians, Chinese, and Indians. Perhaps, suggest many feminists, it is because American society rewards doctors with such prestige and affluence that medicine has remained a near-monopoly for males. At present medical schools are welcoming qualified women candidates, but a true balance still remains distant.

Other grievances include a cynical attitude toward rape, callousness toward the side effects of the birth-control pill ("My doctor said he can live with something as statistically negligible as complications and death from the pill. Well, I can't!"), and a tendency to perform far too many needless hysterectomies and radical mastectomies.

The issue of unnecessary surgery is gaining interest in general. Whereas appendicitis and tonsillectomy are no longer "fashionable" operations, much other surgery, including removal of the gallbladder, is finding its place on operating schedules—whether or not, some critics maintain, it is absolutely necessary.

If it is true that doctors extend better medical care to the affluent than to the impoverished, that they are callous to women and blacks, and cavalier about unneeded surgery, then the coming of the PA may well be the light at the end of the tunnel.

A Human Dimension in Medicine

The career of the PA, coming onto the medical scene without any tradition of dominance by one race or sex, has held out opportunities for all. Blacks and

Hispanics have been with the PA program from its inception. Women, too, have taken their places alongside the men as PAs. This broadly based personnel pool may have the best chance yet to humanize medical care.

So far, most young PAs appear to be intelligent, idealistic, motivated by compassion and concern. The PA can hope to improve his lot, but his labor is not likely to carry him from poverty to riches. There is no conflict of interest between his ideals and the temptation to enrich himself.

The PA is not in a position to recommend surgery of any sort. Being a salaried employee, he has no temptation to pack his waiting room with more patients than can conscientiously be seen in the course of a day. Naturally, there will be pressure periods and patients who must be "worked in somehow," but there should be no deliberate effort to make an already overcrowded afternoon yet more profitable.

A relaxed, receptive attitude toward patients is an important PA attribute. There is no guarantee that no PA anywhere will ever lapse into pride, prejudice, gruffness, or haste—PAs are human, too. But entrants to this new field have been carefully screened and, it is hoped, the unsuitable personalities eliminated. The PA should have the patience to visit thoroughly with each of his patients, to get the whole story in the patient's own words, and to explain in simple phrases exactly what is wrong and what treatment is being prescribed.

The PA need not, of course, be an expert writer or speech maker. But he must be able to communicate with a patient—relating, supporting, encouraging, discussing, reassuring. Language forms a large part of that, but so does nonverbal relating. Warmth and human concern are what the PA can bring to medicine—which will make the ultimate difference in the quality of healing and the quality of life itself.

The prospective PA should ask himself a very important question: Do feelings matter in health care? Do alienation and loneliness, grief and desperation, aging, loss of love, a sense of worthlessness—do these affect the course of ill health and the return of good health? Is failing health worsened because one fails to encounter sympathy, acceptance, and moral support throughout the course of one's treatment? The answer would seem to be yes.

Many reformers look forward to a day when all Americans will be provided with health insurance. The PA should figure prominently in such programs. Widespread use of PAs offers possibilities of extending health care and improving it without bankrupting the nation. Extended health-care programs, in turn, should provide scope for PA leadership and growth.

The PA has yet to be heard from as a professional. To date, the academic physicians, who have been his sponsoring godparents, have explained the PA and defined the role of the PA. The literature concerning the PA movement is doctor-conceived and doctor-written and naturally reflects the doctors' point of view.

It is time for this to change, and it is changing. The professional PA will have to look toward the future and begin to direct the course of his own profession. The *American Academy of Physicians' Assistants, 2341 Jefferson Davis Highway, Arlington, Virginia 22202* (an excellent source of information and literature) has led the drive toward professional independence. PAs are beginning to view themselves as their own persons, not as substitute doctors or extensions of doctors. Perhaps this will truly humanize medical care.

8

IF YOU DON'T MAKE IT AS A PA...

Medical schools, overwhelmed with applications, must reject candidates left and right. But a determined rejectee still has a number of courses open to him. He can go abroad to study in one of Europe's six-year medical schools. He can change to an allied field and become a dentist or a veterinarian or enroll in a combination Ph.D.-M.D. program. One young man, turned down by thirty-three medical schools, joined the Peace Corps and spent two years as the sole public-health official in a primitive African village; this experience so enhanced his candidacy that on his return he was accepted by one of the schools that had previously turned him down.

But what can a rejected PA do? For him, there is no such fine array of alternatives.

Well, first, of course, you can pull yourself together and not give in to a sudden sense of inadequacy. Your rejection has no bearing on your value as a human being; it may not even have a bearing on you as a potential PA. Like the rejected would-be doctor, you are up against a problem of numbers—there are too many applicants for the available places.

Next, consider your options, carefully and fastidiously.

1. You can accept the fact that you have been rejected as "the way things are." There's nothing shameful about that. You made a valiant stab at it and were unsuccessful. Oh, well. Thomas Edison never made it as a scholar, either. So be it. You'll get a job with the phone company.

2. You can declare, at least to yourself, that you won't take it lying down. You made a commitment to becoming a PA. You are going to try again—and again and again if you have to—to get yourself accepted in some PA program.

3. You can switch to another kind of health career. In this burgeoning field, there is a wide choice of careers. Analyze your skills and look around.

Option 1: So Be It.

Most people frustrated in their first career choice settle for something else. If you decide to go this route, it may take some time to adjust.

Take your time to think about a career. You will find that the decision you will finally make about your future will prove to be a solid one because you were not hasty or desperate in making it.

Students often ask for help in vocational decision making, as though there were a *single* career choice for which they were intended. For a Mozart or a Picasso, perhaps so, but most of us can do many things with near-equal effectiveness. Rejection in one career may be only the prologue to a happy, successful life in a quite different and previously unthought-of field.

Option 2: If at First You Don't Succeed . . .

You refuse to take no for an answer. You have applied to, let us say, four PA programs and been turned away by all of them. But, in effect, you reject their rejections. What next?

It is probably too late to send out additional applications for the next admission year. Besides, it is probably pointless. The time has come for careful, objective analysis of your experience.

Perhaps you can do this yourself. It does not hurt, however, to find a good vocational counselor, college teacher, or adviser, someone who can spend a few sessions with you and help you to pinpoint what precisely caused your disappointment.

Was yours a strong application? Take a fresh look at your credentials. (Be honest. This is no time for self-delusion.) After all, it is this very same record, this very same work experience that will be climbing the next stone wall and the next. Try to see yourself as though you were a member of an admissions committee flooded with applicants. How do you look now—one eager candidate among many eager candidates?

Is your educational preparation minimal? Catalog requirements are sometimes stated in terms of the-least-we-will-accept. Are that single year of biology and that single earth-science course all you have behind you? Do you suspect that successful candidates have more impressive educational credits to offer than you do? If so, some extension courses in your areas of weakness may be needed to beef up your record.

What about your experience? When a program emphasizes direct patient-care work experience as an essential of your candidacy, it is wise not to gloss over it and offer a token qualification. "At least a year" probably means "more than a year," never "eight months." "Direct patient-care experience" does not mean as ward clerk or kitchen aide. You may do better by getting more or better experience before reapplying.

What about your references? Were they written by persons who had as much conviction about your future career as you have? Are they interested in you? Do they know what a PA actually is or view the field with prejudice or indifference? Whatever they wrote about you was carefully evaluated. If you think you have been damned with faint praise, you may wish to find new references for your next application.

What about the personal interview? Was it flat? Nervous? Babbling? Did you answer questions of opinion in monosyllables and grunts? Did you keep repeating "y'know" and "y'unnerstand" and "like"? Chew gum throughout the interview? Boast? Belabor the obvious? Try too hard to make an impression? Practice for your next try, working on your rough spots.

Last of all, there an additional step you can take—but, please, only with extreme forethought. You may now legally request to view your file in the PA program's admissions office.

The "right to know" legislation became a thorn in the side of counselors and admissions officers the day it was passed. Among the people who must submit material to college admissions offices, there is so much discomfort over the possibility that once confidential files will be read that many refrain from writing recommendations of any sort. Instead of a candid opinion of the student's potential, they send a "naked" transcript of subjects and grades, leaving unanswered all questions of judgment.

Still, if you are honestly baffled by your rejection and if you have no plans to reapply to that particular program, the right-to-know law may prove valuable. It is not easy or pleasant to read a candid opinion of yourself, but the evaluation, if hard on the ego, should prove educational.

Quite likely you will find the aforementioned thin credentials. The grades may be just so-so, the science preparation minimal, the experience unconvincing, the references lukewarm. If there is some deeper reason, you may need professional guidance as to the best way to handle that.

Fortunately, as we have seen, most of the flaws are remediable. But you must be hard on yourself. There was some once-over-lightly delusion in your first round of application. Do not repeat this costly error.

Option 3: If Not a PA . . .

If your desires for a health career are stronger than your desire to become a PA, you may want to consider an alternative kind of medical career. The satisfaction of knowing that one's lifework is essential to healing others is not limited to doctors and PAs. The qualities in you that attracted you to such a career are applicable to an entire cluster of careers.

Don't stumble helplessly into a consolation-prize career. Allow yourself time to explore the entire field of health care at a level appropriate to your goals. This refers to the years of education required, the difficulty of admission to a training program (all health programs are limited as to the number that can, for laboratory, clinical, or other reasons, be accommodated at one time), and the job outlook.

Research your problem thoroughly, and make sure what you choose is what you can happily spend your life doing. Because many health careers do present open-end and developing opportunities for gainful employment, young people caught up in a depressed economy often plunge into them without really understanding anything except how much money they can ultimately hope to earn. Then they find themselves locked into an irksome or boring career.

"In health careers, it's either love or hate," says Jane Dickinson. She adds, "And it had better be love. . . ."

Here are some of the new and promising careers you might consider:

The *nuclear medicine technologist* works with radioactive isotopes, which are administered to patients for diagnosis and treatment. The AMA describes this technologist as one who "receives, positions and attends to patients and abstracts data from patient records, makes dose calculations . . . and assists the physician in the operation of scanning devices using isotopes. He is greatly concerned with safety and has the responsibility for the disposal of radioactive waste, safe storage of radioactive material, and the inventory and control of radiopharmaceuticals."

Beginning salaries for such technologists are between $10,000 and $11,000 a year.

The *diagnostic medical sonographer* or *ultrasonic technologist* "makes use of sonic energy to determine the contours and composition of body tissues. These procedures make it possible to visualize anatomical, pathological, and functional data to aid the physician in the diagnosis of disease and injury. . . . The sonographer must perform a diagnostic scan and make a permanent record of the significant functional and/or anatomical and pathological data obtained for interpretation by a physician."

Both careers are sophisticated extensions of what used to be called X-ray technology. Starting salaries of both seem comparable, and advancement to $20,000 or more is definitely in sight. Both areas require a background in anatomy, physiology, physics, pathology, and clinical instrumentation. Skills may be acquired on a junior-college level, and although neither program calls for the sustained person-to-person relationships essential to PAs, ability to relate to patients is important.

The field of the *respiratory therapist*, although not new, has grown more complex and specialized of late. This health worker "performs procedures crucial in maintaining life of seriously ill patients with respiratory problems and assists in the treatment of heart and lung ailments, such as cardiac failure, asthma, emphysema, cerebral thrombosis, hemorrhage and shock." This career may also be pursued on a junior-college level. Starting salaries are slightly lower than those received by the other two positions just described. Because training in these areas is expanding, opportunities for advancement should open in teaching or supervisory positions.

Specialist in blood bank technology might offer a fine career to those who enjoy laboratory procedures. And the traditional field, never overcrowded, of *medical record administration* might prove suitable for someone good at details, particularly if it is combined with a knowledge of information-retrieval systems.

The AMA will send, free, single copies of *Education for Allied Medical Careers*, an incomplete, inexpensively prepared, brochure-type compendium valuable mostly for its listing of professional associations or registries where one may write for detailed information concerning health careers and education.

There are, as we have seen, many options for the disappointed. Whether you decide to leave the arena altogether, to try again for an appointment to a PA program, or to seek another equally satisfying health career depends on your temperament, reasoning, and your financial situation, as well as on the availability of opportunities. It is a decision that should be made by you alone, with as much objectivity as you can summon in thinking about your own future.

Useful Addresses:

Accredited programs in all health careers. American Medical Association, 535 North Dearborn Street, Chicago, Illinois 60610. Ask for literature and lists.

Blood Bank Technology. American Society of Clinical Pathologists, P. O. Box 4862, Chicago, Illinois 60680.

Medical Record Administration. American Medical Record Association, 875 North Michigan Avenue, Suite 1850, Chicago, Illinois 60611.

Nuclear Medicine Technology. American Society of Clinical Pathologists, P. O. Box 4862, Chicago, Illinois 60680.

Respiratory Therapy. National Board for Respiratory Therapy, 1900 West 47th Street, Westwood, Kansas 66205.

At present there is no certifying body for *ultrasonic technology.* A nearby teaching hospital is probably the best resource. Address your query to the chief radiologist.

9

LEGAL ASPECTS
OF PA PRACTICE

Do PAs have to pass licensing examinations? Not yet, but there are still legal formalities to be observed by physicians' associates and those who employ them.

The PA arrived on the health scene with such swiftness that a uniformly required and accepted licensing examination has not as yet been entered on all the books. However, twelve states do require PAs to pass either a state or a national certification examination. Success in the latter leads to certification by the National Commission on Certification of PAs. This may aid interstate registration and give the PA freedom to practice almost anywhere. It is not a general must to take this exam, although it may well become one at some time in the near future.

By February, 1978, a total of 5,430 PAs had successfully passed the National Certifying Examination and been awarded the title Physician Assistant-Certified (PA-C).

Regulations Covering PA Practice

Forty-five states have enacted laws concerning the practice of PAs, and these have interesting ramifications. Let us examine a few of these laws.

We have first what the Association of Physician Assistant Programs calls *general delegatory legislation* (also known as *simple authorization statute*). The terms refer to permission given doctors to employ PAs under their supervision and control. Within this type of legislation, the physician has sole responsibility for determining the competence of a PA and deciding what the PA may or may not do in the course of his/her professional activity.

The following states have passed general delegatory legislation pertaining to PAs: Colorado, Connecticut, Delaware, and Tennessee.

Regulatory authority statutes give the state medical licensing board or state health department jurisdiction to pass conditions and regulations concerning PA education and the employment of PAs. This type of legislation covers PA practice in Alabama, Alaska, Arizona, Arkansas, California, Florida, Georgia, Hawaii, Idaho, Illinois, Indiana, Iowa, Kansas, Louisiana, Maine, Maryland, Massachusetts, Michigan, Minnesota, Nebraska, Nevada, New Hampshire, New Mexico, New York, North Carolina, North Dakota, Ohio, Oklahoma, Oregon, Pennsylvania, Rhode Island, South Carolina, South Dakota, Texas, Utah, Vermont, Virginia, Washington, West Virginia, Wisconsin, and Wyoming.

The prevalence of regulatory statutes—those authorizing boards of medical examiners to control the expanded delegation of medical services—has a brief but interesting history.

Late in 1970, when the arrival of the PA was beginning to be noted, the AMA House of Delegates went on record "to remove any barriers to increased delegation of tasks to allied health personnel by physicians." *Allied health personnel* was used in its broadest sense, to include PAs, RNs, and LPNs.

At that time, four states had simple authorization laws; during 1971 and 1972 five more states passed such legislation.

By June 1972 the AMA House of Delegates *reversed itself*, suggesting that licensing boards be set up to approve "on an individual basis" the PA, the supervising doctor, and the description of the job to be performed by the PA. They also recommended that third-party reimbursement (by insurance companies, government agencies, etc.) for medical costs could be made to physicians *for services rendered by PAs supervised by them.* Moreover, such reimbursement was to be limited to services that had prior licensing-board approval.

In a fascinating article in the *Kansas Law Review*, "Physician's Assistant and Nurse Practitioner Laws: a Study of Health Law Reform," Professor C. Kissam of the University of Kansas comments: "One may ask whether the AMA's June 1972 recommendation was not prompted more by an interest in establishing organized medicine's control over expanded medical delegation than in solving a particular reimbursement problem caused by conservative bureaucracies."

Professor Kissam goes on to say, "The physician will be legally responsible for his or her negligence in selecting the non-physician, in selecting the acts to be delegated, and in supervising the non-physician's performance. The physician also will be responsible under the master-servant doctrine for negligent performance by PA . . . employees."

Malpractice

Malpractice is the failure of a professional person to do a professional job, and in the medical profession, it usually means that a doctor has failed to apply the ordinary standards of care to a certain patient's case, the result being injurious to the patient. If it can be proved that a doctor was negligent in a case, he can be sued for a large sum of money.

Most doctors carry insurance against malpractice suits, which have been so successful in recent years and won such enormous settlements from juries sympathetic to patients that the cost of carrying such insurance has risen to unprecedented heights.

Do PAs carry malpractice insurance, too? Most of them do. So do many nurses and other health professionals. According to the Insurance Rating Board, the physician employing a PA pays "a small additional charge" on his own professional liability insurance, which covers his assistant; a PA is assessed approximately half the amount paid by a physician. The cost of such coverage may be the responsibility of the employer or the employing institution. It may be carried independently by the PA.

Geoffrey Francoeur, Jane Dickinson, and Colleen Lemaire are covered by malpractice insurance, the premium for which is paid by their employers, the two hospitals and the health center.

In addition, Colleen carries personal malpractice insurance to supplement the hospital's liability at a cost of a little over ninety dollars a year. "It's not really necessary, but for me it's peace of mind," she said. "In Emergency Service you are often forced to act quickly. I'm only human. There's always the possibility of human error." She feels, moreover, that she owes both herself and the hospital the extra coverage. "The fringe benefits here are so very good—life insurance, hospitalization, accident insurance, even coffee for my coffee breaks—that it seems only decent to carry part of my malpractice insurance."

None of the three knew of an instance where an individual suit had been brought against a PA. "It's bound to happen sooner or later as the public becomes aware of us and what we do," said Jane. "In fact, it's probably happened somewhere."

Geoffrey seems unworried. "Where we're part of a large outfit such as a government hospital, I doubt that anyone would single us out for a lawsuit," he speculated. "Even if negligence was involved, it's lots more profitable to sue Uncle Sam."

How Much Responsibility?

Should PAs make judgments of diagnosis and treatment?

Should PAs practice independently—that is, in a location remote and separate from the supervising physician?

Should PAs write prescriptions for drugs and dispense them?

What, in short, is the scope of a PA's practice? Is there a fine line separating what the PA may and may not do?

All general authorization statutes and some of the regulatory ones leave such questions largely to the discretion of the responsible physicians. Under other regulatory statutes, the scope of practice is resolved on a one-case-at-a-time basis, the determining factor being the particular job description submitted to the medical licensing board.

All of this leaves a vast limbo, beginning with those areas which have, as yet, passed no laws concerning the practice of PAs.

Late in 1971, the AMA's House of Delegates approved the "Essentials of an Approved Educational Program for the Assistant to the Primary Care Physician." These are the accepted standards for training primary-care PAs. The document immediately proclaims that the assistant "will not supplant the doctor in the sphere of decision-making required to establish a diagnosis and plan therapy."

No reason is offered. Professor Kissam comments, "If established by law, this prohibition would help ensure that PAs . . . merely supplement rather than substitute for physicians' services." A possible explanation for the AMA's position is that "supplemental services by PAs . . . are likely to generate a new demand for medical services, thereby protecting physicians' fees and incomes."

The AMA "Essentials," nevertheless, acknowledges the fact that PAs may indeed perform a large range of medical procedures, as well as certain kinds of treatment and emergency diagnosis followed by treatment decisions. They regard such procedures as "executing the physicians' standing orders."

In effect, then, under "standing orders," a PA does indeed determine the severity of symptoms, indicate treatment, and prescribe drugs. And the "Essentials" define the PAs' services as including "independent performance of evaluative and treatment procedures essential to provide an appropriate response to life-threatening emergency situations."

The AMA "Essentials" make no mention of "remote" practice (in a site other than the supervising physician's) or drug dispensation. There is, however, a general statement that practice variations may result from "geographic, economic, and sociologic factors." Professor Kissam indicates that "the recognition of the execution of standing orders . . . seems to imply authority to engage in limited, independent decision-making with respect to drugs."

Most state laws do not spell out boundaries as to what a PA may or may not do. Some states (Nevada and Washington are examples) do allow PAs to make diagnostic and treatment judgments. About half the regulatory statutes permit "acts of medical diagnosis" and "prescription of medical, therapeutic, or corrective measures." The majority of states are ambiguous and some have, to date, no legislation whatsoever pertaining to the licensing, training, and employment of PAs or what they are permitted to do.

Hospitals are especially vulnerable to lawsuits. What about the employment of PAs by hospitals or health-care centers?

New York's Health Department has perhaps been the most active and aware in its supervision of institutional medical care. Its regulations appear to encourage extended participation in health-care institutions (which would include hospitals, nursing homes, and health-care centers). A physician is allowed to supervise a maximum of six PAs employed by such an institution. This makes it possible for New York hospital physicians to make much greater use of PAs than those in most other states, where an institutional doctor may be restricted to one or two.

New York regulations, moreover, expressly permit PAs employed by institutions to dispense drugs to inpatients, if the medical orders are countersigned by the supervising physician within twenty-four hours. This is a more liberal practice than prevails in most states, which are either more restrictive or totally silent on this issue.

Under the regulations of thirteen or more states, PAs must be employed by physicians only or by physician-owned corporations. In other words, there exists some prohibition against the employment of PAs by hospitals. This is a narrow interpretation of the AMA's very guarded and carefully phrased "Essentials," perhaps based on a fear that, if a hospital administration, rather than a doctor, is responsible for the hiring, firing, and general supervision of the PA, the employment of such nondoctors would escape the doctors' control.

In actuality, hospitals are interested in the expanded use of PAs for dollars-and-cents reasons primarily. Where such utilization has been accomplished, the expansion of outpatient and emergency services would seem to prove the wisdom of such procedures. Professor Kissam feels that restricting hospital employment of PAs—ostensibly to protect the public—actually just limits the use of PAs to areas where they will not provide a threat to physicians' and nurses' income and practice.

As for the supervision of PAs by doctors in private practice, twenty-one states limit a doctor to one or two—although waivers of this limitation have gone on record in three of these states. Most laws are not explicit concerning numbers. New York authorizes a maximum of four in private practice, six in a hospital setting. Maryland allows two in "noninstitutional practice," an undisclosed larger number in institutional settings. Wisconsin and New Mexico permit the supervision of two PAs, with medical boards able to grant waivers permitting a larger number. New Mexico also permits PA "teams"—but only for free medical services.

What's Ahead?

What can the young PA hope for in the future, with respect to the legal structure of his profession? PA practitioners are quite outspoken about what they want.

1. They are in favor of state or national licensure by examination and believe such an examination will be a

requirement for certification in the future. "After all, doctors and nurses have to take qualifying exams," says Geoffrey Francoeur. "I think such an examination would prove that we, too, have a body of knowledge."

2. Legal authorization for the PA to diagnose and prescribe whatever therapy (including medication and drugs) might be indicated in accordance with the policies of the supervising physician but *not* requiring blow-by-blow sanction. "Either we are professionals or we are not," says Colleen Lemaire.

3. Authorization to practice in any medical setting: hospital, health-care center, nursing home, private office.

4. Explicit authorization to practice in remote locations. ("That means away from the supervising doctor and that has to mean a PA in private practice. . . .")

5. Clear definition of scope of practice. ("They've got to make up their minds, legally, what we may and may not do.")

6. More uniformity in PA programs of study.

7. Credit toward the M.D. degree in medical schools. ("I can't understand this closed-shop attitude," says Jane. "I think what PAs have is medical preparation—don't you?")

Obviously the degree of independent responsibility permitted a PA has yet to be established. These are surely the next steps in the development of the newest and most promising health career.

10

PAs, NURSES, AND NURSE PRACTITIONERS

At about the time the PA movement was born and began to make a lasting impression, nursing, too, started to examine its education and role with a view to extending the scope of that profession.

What emerged was the *nurse practitioner*, a fully trained registered nurse with additional postgraduate study in diagnosis and treatment of patients.

From the very start of their side-by-side existence, PAs and NPs have been compared and contrasted, challenged and disputed. They have viewed one another as friend or foe, excited partisans and detractors, and confused many of us as to where they are alike and where different.

There is reason for the confusion. PAs and nurses, after all, are both highly skilled and carefully schooled members of the health team, second in knowledge and skill only to the physician. And because both professions are engaged in patient care, there is inevitable overlapping.

Geoffrey Francoeur, Jane Dickinson, and Colleen Lemaire believe the PA has a more responsible role in health care than a nurse. "The PA *performs* where the nurse *assists*," said Geoffrey. "When I worked in the emergency room, I could examine the patient, order X rays, locate the problem, and set the broken bone—all in the time it takes a nurse to find out what the doctor wants."

"Not if the nurse is a practitioner," Jane admitted. "I agree the PA does some things a nurse practitioner doesn't—like suturing and casting. But there's really very little difference."

"Oh, if it's an NP, there's practically none."

At the health-care center where Jane works, some departments employ a PA and others an NP. The team roles are comparable, the salaries the same. "Some departments prefer NPs," she says. "Pediatrics, for one. And obstetrics. We have a super nurse-midwife."

The very term "nurse-midwife" is a reminder of possibly the oldest kind of health career. But today's educated nurse-midwife bears little resemblance to the raw-knuckled neighbor called in "when the time came" in towns and villages the world over. She is a sophisticated, medically knowledgeable expert, certified by official examination, who is prepared not only to deliver babies but to teach prospective parents to participate jointly in the experience of birth.

The training of a nurse practitioner, which comes

after completion of the nursing course (although changes are contemplated), is usually shorter than that of PA. Certificate courses range from six to eight weeks to a year, with most programs approximately a year in length. Practitioner programs may be part of degree programs, although usually they are not.

Why does it take so much less time to train a nurse practitioner than a PA? Because the starting point is the educated nurse. PAs, like beginning medical students, may have a good science background, but in the area of patient care they are literally starting from scratch.

The student looking ahead to a career in health care should consider numerous possibilities, some of which he or she will reject while finding others worthy of consideration. Since the PA and NP are professionals closely aligned in function, and since many of their tasks are identical, they deserve a long look in relation to one another.

Which Is Which?

The NP is part of an old profession with its own tradition and literature.

The PA is a pathfinder, too new to have a real professional tradition, still engaged in defining his/her role and identity.

All registered nurses must be licensed by their states. Licensing examinations are encouraged by most PA programs, but are not mandatory in all states. This, too, may change. By early 1977 approximately 4,500 graduate PAs had successfully passed the examination given by the National Board of Medical Examiners of the Washington-based American Academy of Physician's Assistants.

NPs see themselves as accountable only to their own profession. The PA does not agree, viewing *both* professions accountable to the hospital, physician, or health-care center which employs them.

What about the economics of these professions?

Although staff salaries are comparable, an odd situation has developed with respect to opportunities. As a newcomer to the health-care field, the PA finds entry-level positions more numerous. The new PA is in the enviable situation of being sought out by prospective employers.

The NP, however, sees more room at the top. Because nursing is an old profession, it has developed every type of leadership—administrative, teaching, research. A nurse or NP may go on to a master's or a doctor's degree and a highly rewarding leadership career. There are some NPs with academic rank who teach medical students.

There is little doubt that the PA will, with time and widespread acceptance, develop leadership opportunities. For the time being, the view from the bottom looks very good indeed.

Pulling It Together

The PA and the NP should enjoy a complementary, rather than a competitive, relationship, and in places where they work side by side, they usually do.

The world needs good health-care practitioners, whether their name is NP or PA. With a burgeoning population of senior citizens, an increase in deaths from cancer and heart attacks, ignorance concerning the toxic residues of civilization, birth defects, and the psychobiological havoc that attends the stresses of our time, we need all the help available.

APPENDIX A: PROGRAMS OF VARYING LENGTHS

Some General Procedures

Unlike the college-bound high-school senior who has access to counselors, data banks, agencies, and advisory committees, the PA candidate is often totally without guidance.

The field is relatively new, and the programs are geographically scattered, differing in length and sometimes in scope. As a consequence, some counselors are still unaware of this health career, and many more, though aware of it, are only sketchily informed. Few, as yet, have had extensive personal contact with PAs.

The aspiring PA is urged to embark on an information hunt. He should forage in library reference rooms, speak with doctors, nurses, and other health workers, direct inquiries to personnel officers of hospitals. And no matter where the prospective candidate finds himself, a useful address to bear in mind is that of the professional organization:

> Association of Physician Assistant Programs
> 2120 L Street N. W.
> Washington, D. C.

For a token sum, the association will supply up-to-date essential information.

The search will eventually lead you to practitioners in the field. Ask questions, no matter how naive and elementary. The answers will help you decide what kind of program you should enroll in.

The one question you should *not* ask is "Which is the best PA program?" No school, college, or PA program is indisputably the best. The virtue or value of every judgment is its relationship to someone. No one can predict with certainty that success or failure will inevitably follow a particular step. The wise adviser is strong with information and shy with advice. He will tell you what each particular program consists of and let you choose the one that seems to suit you.

There is disagreement among medical educators as to the way a PA should be trained, the extent of the education, and the length of time necessary to equip a student with or without previous patient-care experience. Consequently, all programs are being constantly changed, improved upon, and reevaluated.

Most PA programs are approximately two years in length and of Type A—preparing a student to assist the primary-care physician. The exceptions are worth studying and evaluating, however. Some of the shorter programs are directed toward specific goals.

At the beginning of the PA movement, all programs awarded a certificate of completion. Many have continued to do so; others have recognized the advantage and the market value of a degree. In the future, all programs may award a bachelor's or a master's degree.

MEDEX Programs

The MEDEX-type programs covered in this section emphasize clinical preparation. The basic sciences and preclinical subjects are usually streamlined within a five-month period in place of the nine to twelve months of the two-year curricula. The clinical phase of the MEDEX program may be less varied. There may be fewer clinical clerkships; a large part of practical training may involve a single block of experience, a preceptorship, under a single, private physician. Frequently this preceptor agrees in advance to employ the student at the end of the period of training. The system has both advantages and limitations.

A few words about the terms "Medex" and "MEDEX." The former, Medex or *a* Medex, describes a PA practitioner; the latter (in capitals) is the educational program. MEDEX programs are AMA-approved.

MEDEX/PA Program, Drew Postgraduate Medical School, 1621 East 120 Street, Los Angeles, California 90059. Fifteen months in length, this program starts

with five months' basic education in clinical and laboratory procedures. This is followed by six months' clinical
experience in maternal-child health, emergency medicine and surgery, and psychiatry. The final phase is a
four-month preceptorship in the office of a private
physician.

High-school graduation and a minimum of sixty
semester hours of college work are required for admission, as is the ACT. Committed to the training of health
practitioners for urban communities, the program
literature emphatically states, "Black and Mexican-
American students are generally in the majority, and at
least one-third of the class are women."

A certificate is awarded. Eligible candidates may
be granted either a B.A. or a B.S. degree by an affiliated college. Tuition is $410 for Californians, $3,000
for nonresidents; approximately $700 is indicated for
equipment and books.

*Physician Assistant Program, Northeastern Univer-
sity, Boston, Massachusetts 02115.* This eighteen-month
program is open to persons who have completed a
minimum of two years of college, including courses in
cell biology and chemistry, and who have had at least a
year of patient-care experience.

One third of the program is "didactic"—i.e., classroom and laboratory studies—including medical laboratory science, interviewing techniques, human anatomy,
physiology, medicine, pediatrics, obstetrics and
gynecology, psychiatry, surgery, rehabilitation, medicine, pharmacology, radiology, electrocardiology, patient education, and PA seminar.

Twelve-week rotations are provided in medicine,

pediatrics, and emergency care, with six-week rotations in mental health, obstetrics, and each of several surgical subspecialties. Academic credit is given.

Tuition and fees total $700 a quarter, offset by federal funds. Books and equipment total approximately $300.

The Physician's Assistant Program, Pennsylvania State University, formerly *MEDEX /Pennsylvania, Milton S. Hershey Medical Center, Hershey, Pennsylvania 17033*, is an eighteen-month program under the direction of the College of Medicine of Pennsylvania State University. Applicants should be high-school graduates, should have had three years of patient-care experience involving at least fourteen weeks of formal training, and indicate their willingness to live and work in the mid-Atlantic region served by the program. Applicants are initially screened by the MEDEX staff, with the final selection made by the group of physician-preceptors with whom they will be associated.

The preclinical phase of five months' duration is conducted at the medical center at Hershey. The final ten months are spent with the participating physician. The program is very intensive and involves relocation in central Pennsylvania.

Tuition is $460 a term for residents, $916 for non-residents. Textbooks and miscellaneous equipment total about $300.

MEDEX Physician's Assistant Program, Medical University of South Carolina, Charleston, South Carolina 29401. This is a twelve-month program for college graduates with a strong biological sciences background or a combination of college education and patient-care experience.

The university phase of the program, covering two quarters, emphasizes medical history, diagnostic skills, and "human relations and personality studies." The final two quarters are spent in a clinical preceptorship under the close supervision of a practicing physician. The location of the preceptorship may be at a considerable distance from the university; academic ties will continue, with travel expenses the responsibility of the student.

A tuition fee of $880 has been charged residents, with nonresidents of South Carolina paying $1,760. Books, equipment and health fees total $350. A certificate and fifty-five quarter hours of academic credit are earned.

Utah MEDEX Project, University of Utah Medical Center, 50 North Medical Drive, Salt Lake City, Utah 84132, is a twelve-month program without higher-education requirements but open only to persons with approximately three years of patient-related medical experience in either a civilian or a military setting. The project has as an objective preparing practitioners for rural and medically underserved areas.

It is unique in that the physician preceptors are known in advance. The student is carefully assigned to his preceptor, who supervises his training and is committed to employ the student after graduation. Of course, the student's training is geared to the preceptor's practice. The Medex trainee is thereby assured of a practice when training is completed; he is by that time thoroughly familiar with that practice.

The first four to five months are in a medical-center setting and consist of lectures, demonstrations, and clinical work. The preceptorship phase of seven to eight months is spent within an eight-state Intermountain Region with the practice of the physician-preceptor. During this period trainees are required to return periodically to the Medical Center in Salt Lake City for evaluation and continuing instruction.

A certificate is awarded; fifty quarter hours of college credit may be earned. There is no charge for tuition; fees are $350.

MEDEX Northwest Program, Department of Health Services, 1107 N. E. 45th Street, Seattle, Washington 98105, is flexible as to time, involving between twelve and sixteen months of study. Begun in response to areas suffering from a shortage of primary-health-care physicians, this program was the first of the MEDEX offerings in the nation and is affiliated with the School of Public Health and Community Medicine of the University of Washington. Endorsed by the Washington State Medical Association, it has cooperative relationships with the medical associations of Alaska, Oregon, Idaho, and Montana.

The instruction is individualized, accounting for differences in completion time. The first five months of instruction involve basic clinical skills: history taking, physical examinations, behavioral skills, and basic technical tasks such as suturing and casting. A special study of child growth and development and experience in emergency care complete this segment of the program. It is followed by an eight-to-twelve-month on-the-job training session in a preceptorship. Evaluation is continued by the MEDEX staff, as well as by the preceptor.

Applicants must have two years' experience in patient care. There are no formal educational requirements beyond high school. Students must indicate a willingness to relocate in the Pacific Northwest.

A certificate is awarded at the conclusion of the program. Tuition is $3,200, with in-state students being charged $916. Books and supplies average $450.

PA Programs Sponsored by the Armed Services

There are two programs open to persons of both sexes who are already on active duty. One of these is operated jointly by the navy and the air force. This is the *School of Health Care Sciences, USAF, Department of Medicine, PA Program, Sheppard AFB, Texas 76311.* The twenty-four-month program involves a tightly packed period of didactic and clinical laboratory education, with the second year consisting of ten rotations offering some elective options. The clinical year (the second) is spent in various air-force and naval hospitals.

Standards are high. Previous school, college, and military performance are factors, as well as above-average grades on standardized examinations, military and premilitary. An arrangement with the University of Nebraska offers ninety semester hours of college credit toward the 130 units required for the B.S. degree. Full military pay and allowances continue throughout the training period. There is, of course, no charge for tuition.

Requirements are somewhat more precisely spelled out for the *U. S. Army Physicians' Assistant Program, Academy of Health Sciences, Fort Sam Houston, Texas 78234*. A high-school diploma or its equivalent, a sound working knowledge of English, a minimum of twenty-four months' duty in a medical military occupational specialty, and qualifications for warrant officer appointment are among the requirements. A pledge of intent to reenlist is also required.

Successful graduates of the program are granted an A.B. degree by Baylor University. A MOS 911A (Military Physicians' Assistant) is also awarded, together with appointment as warrant officer. An active-duty commitment of four years is required.

The two military-service-sponsored programs are among the nation's largest, since they are not limited to one class a year. The combined USAF/USN program accepts 64 students every four months, a total of 192 per year, an impressive number. The clinical year involves the cooperation of 230 supervising physicians, in addition to the 45 doctors and scientists retained for the classroom and laboratory education of the first year.

Programs Accepting Students Directly from High School

These programs exist, but the possibilities are limited. We refer now to programs for students without prior college courses *or* extensive patient-care experience.

The *Physician's Assistant Program, Lake Erie College, 391 West Washington Street, Painesville, Ohio 44077*, incorporates PA training within a four-year women's liberal arts college.

For the first three years students attend Lake Erie College, taking courses, practicums, and internships, and fulfilling the requirements for a B.A. degree. The final year they spend at the Cleveland Clinic Foundation, learning a variety of medical skills.

To be accepted at the clinic, an applicant must be a student in good standing at Lake Erie College and have completed six courses (including biology and chemistry), plus a PA seminar. Graduates are awarded a B.A. degree by Lake Erie College and a certificate by the Cleveland Clinic Educational Foundation.

Tuition is $3,100 for an Ohio resident, $198 per course for a nonresident.

A program of interest to students completing high school is now offered by *St. Francis College, Loretto, Pennsylvania 15940*. High-quality achievement in high-school science courses is essential, as are strong SAT or ACT scores. The first two years of the four-year program will be spent on the St. Francis College campus. During this time, basic sciences and a liberal-arts background of English, history, mathematics, psychology, sociology, and philosophy will be acquired.

The third year will consist of physician-taught classroom work in biomedical physics, diagnostic procedures, anatomy, physiology, pharmacology, public health, and pathology, and the fourth year will be spent in clinical medicine. A B.S. degree will be earned.

Tuition is $75 per credit plus an additional surcharge of $1,000. An additional $300 is needed for books and equipment.

The *Physician's Assistant Program* of *Alderson-Broaddus College, Philippi, West Virginia 26416*, the oldest and best established of the straight-from-high-school PA programs, offers a forty-two-month course sequence leading to the B.S. degree. General education based on the liberal arts and sciences, with numerous options, is carried on concurrently with medical and surgical studies and a variety of clinical experiences in many settings.

Spread throughout a four-year period are core courses in the sciences and basic PA skills. Clinical rotations include medicine, surgery, intensive care, emergency care, and working in a private physician's office. Medical affiliations include institutions in West Virginia, Ohio, South Carolina and the District of Columbia.

Standards are high, with better than average SATs or ACTs required, as well as rank in the upper two -fifths of the candidates' high-school graduating class.

Tuition and fees total $2,468, with about $300 needed for books. Graduates of the four-year program are awarded a B.S. degree with a major in medical science.

Programs Geared to Medical Specialization

The *Surgeon's Assistant Program* of the *School of Medicine, University of Alabama, Birmingham, Alabama 35294*, is a twenty-three-month course emphasizing skills helpful to the surgeon before, during, and after surgery, including operating room, recovery room, intensive care, outpatient clinic, and surgeon's office. Four academic quarters of preclinical course work are followed by thirteen months of clinical education. A variety of surgical services are explored, each for a six-week period.

Entrance requirements call for sixty semester hours of college, including at least one year of general biology and one year of general chemistry. Other sciences are specifically recommended. High-school and college work must be of high caliber.

A B.S. degree is awarded. Tuition is $1,700 for an Alabama resident, $3,400 for a nonresident, with books and equipment estimated at $500.

The *Child Health Program* of the *University of Colorado Medical Center, 4200 East 9th Avenue, Denver 80220*, emphasizes the comprehensive health care of children through adolescence. The handbook states, "Graduates . . . are qualified to diagnose, treat, and manage most of the common medical and psychosocial problems of childhood and adolescence. . . . Graduates are able to care for approximately 80 percent of the patients seen in a typical pediatric practice."

The first year of the thirty-three-month curriculum emphasizes the basic sciences, history taking, diagnosis. Clinical experience in the baby clinic, newborn nursery, and pediatric hospital wards begins early in the program. Half the second year involves pharmacology, emergency practice, psychosomatic and emotional problems, and child development, with the other half spent in pediatric rotations. A year of internship follows.

Sixty semester hours of college credits, with year-long courses in chemistry, biology, and psychology plus a humanities course, are required for admission. At the end of the second year a B.S. degree in child-health associate is awarded. The M.S. degree may be earned by students whose credentials meet graduate-school requirements.

Tuition and fees are $1,208 for a Colorado resident and $4,835 for a nonresident, with $420 indicated in miscellaneous fees.

The *Physician's Assistant in Pathology Program* of the *School of Allied Health and Natural Sciences, Quinnipiac College, Hamden, Connecticut 06518* offers a unique two-year, two-summer course to qualified candidates who already hold a bachelor's degree.

The program trains students to assist in the performance of postmortem and surgical specimen examinations, to dictate autopsy findings and the dissection of specimen descriptions, and to assume administrative and supervisory responsibilities over a morgue, tissue storage and surgical dissection areas, laboratory photography section, and histology, cytology and clerical personnel.

The program is offered in conjunction with Yale University School of Medicine, a nearby Veteran's Administration hospital, and other Connecticut facilities.

Applicants must have an appropriate science background which should include courses in organic chemistry, biochemistry and/or quantitative analysis. A grade point average of at least 2.5 is required.

Tuition is $75 per semester hour of credit; there are miscellaneous fees. At the successful conclusion of the program a Master of Science degree is awarded.

To enter the *Surgeon's Assistant Program of the University of North Carolina, Chapel Hill 27514,* a candidate must have high SAT or ACT scores, two years of college-level work and two years of patient-care experience. Communication skills are important.

The initial eight months of didactic classroom instruction covers blood-banking, operating-room techniques, basic sciences, asepsis, histories and physical examinations, EKG, medical electronic equipment, X-ray interpretation. During the following sixteen months of clinical training the student gains experience in most medical specialties.

A total of $800 covers tuition, fees, books, and equipment. A certificate is awarded.

I have omitted a description of the *MEDEX/Pacific Program* of the *University of Hawaii,* open only to graduate nurses from Micronesia and established for the purpose of providing medical practitioners from the Trust Territory of the Pacific Islands.

APPENDIX B:
TWO-YEAR COURSES

By far the largest number of PA practitioner programs are approximately two years in length and have as their goal the training of assistants to primary-care physicians.

They differ in emphasis. Some require substantial experience in patient health care, others prefer academic background, some demand both. From year to year, searching revaluations by the leadership of the programs may bring about sweeping changes.

The *Primary Care Associate Program* of *Stanford University Medical Center, Palo Alto, California 94304,* is a joint program of that center and several community colleges located in a predominantly agricultural area of the state.

During the first nine-month academic year, students

remain at their respective junior colleges for a sequence of basic science courses and an introduction to primary care. This is followed by a full calendar year at the health center and its clinical facilities. The last five months involve a preceptorship served under a physician in family practice. An A.S. degree and a certificate are awarded.

The program is offered to high-school graduates with a distinguished record and a strong science preparation, together with "a significant degree of responsible health-care experience." Tuition is a token $20 for Californians. Nonresidents are charged $26 a credit.

The *Physician Associate Program, Yale University School of Medicine, 333 Cedar Street, New Haven, Connecticut 06510,* is a twenty-four-month program to train "advanced health care practitioners." PA students take many basic courses alongside regular medical-school students and candidates for advanced degrees in nursing, medical sciences, and public health. Broad social goals, a humanistic approach to science, and a high degree of medical knowledge and skills are among the objectives of the program.

A nine-month period of lectures and laboratories is followed by fifteen months of five-week rotations in most branches of medicine and medical specialties. A limited number of these, occurring at the end of the program, are elective. A certificate is awarded.

Two years of college with some science emphasis is required for admission; applicants with a baccalaureate degree are given preference. Character references, SAT scores, and direct patient-care experience are also factors.

Tuition is $2,900 per annum, with approximately $500 cited for books and equipment.

George Washington University's School of Medicine and Health Sciences, Washington, D.C. 20037, offers a twenty-four-month Physician Assistant Program. Forty-six semester hours of preclinical courses comprise the first year: chemistry, anatomy and physiology, human behavior, physical diagnosis, pharmacology, clinical pathology, medicine, animal surgery, electrocardiography, introduction to radiology, related courses. The second year is comprised of clinical rotations in a variety of services.

For admission a candidate must meet the requirements of the university and present a minimum of one year of health-related training, either civilian or military. Exceptions may be made with respect to this requirement. Certification is earned by all who successfully complete the program. Those who present or acquire an additional thirty hours of credit in the humanities, mathematics, and/or the social sciences may be awarded a B.S. degree by the School of Medicine and Health Sciences.

Tuition and fees total $4,360, with books and equipment estimated at $500.

In 1977 the *PA/MEDEX Program, Howard University, 6th and Bryant Streets N. W., Washington, D.C. 20059* changed its curriculum from fifteen months to twenty-four months without a change of name.

The first year is devoted to instruction in the basic health sciences. The student then spends a month each in clinical medicine, surgery, pediatrics, obstetrics and gynecology, psychiatry, ambulatory care, and emergency service. The final semester is a preceptorship, with the student working under a primary-care physician in private practice. It is possible to earn ninety-four college credits toward the B.S. within the program.

The Howard MEDEX program places great emphasis on previous health experience and seeks applicants from those with military medical training, RNs, LPNs, and other health workers. Tuition and fees total $1,854, with $800 earmarked for books and equipment and $36 for insurance.

The *Physician's Assistant Program* of the *College of Medicine, University of Florida, Gainesville, Florida 32610,* offers a twenty-four month course leading to a B.S. degree in medicine. The faculty of this institution, as well as guest lecturers, collaborate in the course work, with the clinical portion of the program coordinated by the Department of Community Health of the University of Florida.

Admission requirements call for one year's experience in patient care and two year's credits toward a bachelor's degree (preferably in the science area). Instrumentation, patient evaluation, minor surgery, pharmacology, pediatrics, obstetrics, and gynecology are included in the clinical courses, as are internships and preceptorships.

Students who are residents of Florida pay $16.50 a credit in tuition and fees, and nonresidents are assessed $51.50 a credit. Books and equipment are budgeted at $700.

The *Physician Associate Program, Division of Allied Health Professions, Emory University, Atlanta, Georgia 30322*, requires twenty-seven months, the classroom and clinical portions followed by a terminal practicum for some students. Undergraduate science makes up the first quarter, followed by four quarters of basic health sciences; and a six-month clinical science core is followed by a six-month "concentration" period. Concentrations are in family practice and primary care. This period allows considerably flexibility as to types of medical setting.

A high-school diploma and satisfactory SAT scores are required of candidates who have not attended college. Health experience is advantageous, though not mandatory. Students completing the course of study are awarded the Associate in Medical Science degree and may go on to earn the B.S. degree.

Tuition and fees total $4,600, with another $500 estimated for books and equipment.

The *Physician Assistants Program* of the *Medical College of Georgia, Augusta 30902*, offers a twenty-four-month program as a department of the School of Allied Health Sciences. The curriculum is divided into three phases: the first on the campus of the college, the second in hospital clinics, and the third in offices and clinics of primary-care physicians.

One must present ninety quarter hours of college work (with science emphasis) for admission. A B.S. degree is awarded.

As in most state institutions and those receiving state subsidies, tuition and fees are higher here (by $448) for nonresidents than for Georgians, who pay $820. Approximately $875 is needed for books and equipment.

The *Physician's Assistant Program* of the *College of Medicine, University of Iowa, Iowa City 52242*, has an admissions requirement of two years of college study, with a strong record in science courses and a grade-point average of at least 2.5. This twenty-four-month program involves three phases, the first didactic, the second a "bridge" to clinical medicine called "Introduction to Clinical Medicine for Physician's Assistant Students," formulated to develop basic skills in history-taking, diagnosis, and interviewing. The third consists of clinical rotations.

Nonresidents of Iowa pay $2,625 in tuition and fees; residents, $1,125. Books, uniforms, and equipment total $400.

Wichita State University, 5500 E. Kellogg Street, Wichita 67218, has a 24-month *Physician's Assistant Program* open to applicants who have either a baccalaureate degree *or* three years of direct patient care experience experience *or* an equivalent combination of both. The first eleven months are didactic, the following thirteen spent in required and elective clinical rotations.

The course leads to certification. Tuition for a Kansas resident is $904, for a nonresident $2,143. Books and equipment total $475.

Clinical Associate Program, College of Allied Health Professions, University of Kentucky, Lexington 40506 admits students with at least two years of college and high scores on scholastic aptitude tests.

The twenty-four-month program is innovative. The first nine months offer an integrated basic science/medical science self-study unit utilizing small-group format, with weekly "plenary sessions." Bedside teaching begins early and is coordinated with each body system studied. Students are able, as a result, to demonstrate acceptable diagnostic techniques before beginning their second, or clinical, year.

Resident tuition is $700; nonresident, $2,070, with $300 suggested for books and equipment.

The *Health Associate Program* of the *Johns Hopkins University School of Health Services, Baltimore, Maryland 21205*, is a twenty-one-month program providing the third and fourth college years and leading to a B.S. degree. Biology, chemistry, mathematics, psychology, and social-science courses are required for admission. The program runs for two academic years, with an intervening ten-week summer session.

In keeping with the Johns Hopkins philosophy and reflected in other schools of the university, lectures, seminars, sciences, humanities, laboratory, and clinical practicum are offered simultaneously, with greater emphasis and more time devoted to clinical practicum throughout the senior year. The program is integrated and interdisciplinary in every sense, organized within a series of units called modules, each of which focuses on a specific area of health care. Both urban and rural health settings are provided for the clinical experience.

Tuition and fees are $3,600 for the nine-month yer, with books and suplies $325. A personal budget of $850 is suggested by the program.

Affiliated with Johns Hopkins and other outstanding hospitals is the twenty-four-month *Physician's Assistant Program* at the *Essex Community College, 7201 Rossville Blvd., Baltimore 21237.* It is directed toward the high-school graduate with considerable health-care experience. Clinical options are available in family practice or public health. An Associate in Arts degree is awarded.

For this program Baltimore County residents are charged $18 a credit, other Maryland residents $36 a credit, and nonresidents $80 a credit, with $200 estimated for books and equipment.

The *Physician's Assistant Program, Mercy College, Detroit, Michigan 28219,* offers a twenty-four-month program within a liberal-arts context. A calendar year is devoted to basic and medical sciences. The second year consists of clinical rotations supplemented by seminars in selected and clinical topics. The course culminates in an eight-week preceptorship in the office of a private practicing physician. At its conclusion a Bachelor of Science degree is awarded.

At least a year of college work with the usual biological and physical-science courses are required for entrance, as well as two or more years of acceptable direct patient experience. Applications from ex-corpsmen, LPNs, RNs, operating-room technicians, and other health personnel are welcome.

Tuition and fees are $2,790, with separate science and clinical course fees (total unstipulated). Books and equipment total $425; health insurance ranges from $50 to $160.

A *Physician's Assistants Program* is offered at *West-*

ern Michigan University, Kalamazoo, Michigan 49008.
This is a transfer program; applicants are required to
have completed sixty semester hours of college credit
with concentration in the sciences. At least one year of
patient contact experience is mandatory. The university
awards a B.S. degree in medicine.

While clinical exposure is offered during the first
phase, basic medical sciences and diagnosis are em-
phasized. The second year consists of clinical rotations in
medicine, surgery, obstetrics and gynecology, pediatrics, psychiatry, and primary care, supplemented by
clinical lectures in these specialties and in dermatology
and allergy.

Tuition and fees total $2,676 for residents, $6,237
for nonresidents, and, for equipment and books, $700.

The *Physician's Assistant Program, St. Louis University Medical Center, St. Louis, Missouri 63104,* is a
twenty-four-month course offered jointly by Washington University School of Medicine and St. Louis University.

Courses in the basic medical sciences, human
dynamics, and comprehensive health care make up the
first phase. Rotating clinical blocks, including both
general surgery and surgical subspecialties, follow. The
final phase is a twenty-week preceptorship.

One year of patient-care experience and two years
of college are required for admission. ACT scores are
mandatory. A certificate is awarded.

The catalog indicates that $3,600 is needed for tui-
tion and other school expenses.

The *Physician's Assistant Program* of the *University of Nebraska Medical Center, Omaha 68105*, is open to students who have completed two years of college and successfully passed courses in English, mathematics, biological science, chemistry, psychology, and electives from the humanities and the social sciences. SAT or ACT is required. A B.S. degree is awarded.

In addition to the didactic and clinical aspects of the program, a sixteen-week period is spent with a rural family practitioner. The stated objectives of the Nebraska program include training assistants for rural practitioners.

Residents pay $1,140 in tuition and fees, nonresidents $2,970. Books and equipment cost $600.

The twenty-four-month *Albany-Hudson Valley Physician's Associate Program, Albany Medical College of Union University, New Scotland Avenue, Albany, New York 12208*, also offers a course of study divided into three phases: the first devoted to the liberal arts and basic sciences at Hudson Valley Community College; the second providing training in "clinical sciences and medical arts" at Albany College of Medicine; the third "enhances clinical proficiency by giving each student a structured medical experience under the supervision and direction of practicing physicians."

High-school graduates with a minimum of *six months'* experience (or 2,000 hours) in patient-care may apply; the SAT is waived only if the candidate is a college graduate. The desire to work in a rural or an inner-city environment will be viewed as a definite plus with respect to admission.

Tuition and fees total $1,237 for a resident, $2,36͡

for an out-of-state resident. Books and equipment cost $450.

An Associate in Applied Science degree from Hudson Valley Community College and a Physician's Associate Certificate from Albany Medical College are awarded.

The *Physician's Assistant Program* of *The Brooklyn Hospital, 121 DeKalb Avenue, Brooklyn, New York,* offers a twenty-two month program in conjunction with the Long Island University and the Brooklyn-Cumberland Medical Center. It is open to juniors at Long Island University or to students who transfer to that university and are accepted into the program.

Classes in English composition, psychology, human sexuality, mathematics, principles of medical science, and anatomy-physiology are held at the New York School of Social Research during the first nine months. A three-month preclinical period, which includes classes in pathology, pharmacology, history taking, physical diagnosis, and clinical techniques and procedures, follows. The final, clinical phase centers around a rotating internship in medicine, neurology, surgery, rehabilitation medicine, anesthesia, inhalation medicine, obstetrics-gynecology, pediatrics, psychiatry, and emergency service. Tuition is $90 per credit plus a $12 fee; books and equipment $250. A B.S. degree is earned.

The Physician's Assistant Program, Harlem Hospital Center, 135th Street and Lenox Avenue, New York, New York 10027, was founded to improve the quality of health care for the black, medically indigent, inner-city resident, but has broaded its basis to train for service to small towns and rural areas as well.

The twenty-eight-month curriculum is divided into three parts, the first of which, the academic phase of nine months, involves general education and a needed science background. The preclinical phase includes pathology, behavioral sciences, biochemistry, pharmacology, history taking, and physical diagnosis, clinical techniques and procedures. This is followed by a twelve-month clinical phase including hospital rotations and a one-to-one preceptorship with a physician in private practice.

There is a $400 charge for tuition, with about $175 needed for books and equipment. Some stipends are available. Approximately 90 percent of the student body, to date, has consisted of minority groups. Out-of-state applicants will be considered only if a firm commitment to return to the home state for practice is demonstrated. Applicants with two years of college and a strong record in the sciences are preferred. Graduates earn a Bachelor of Science degree in health care, awarded by The City College of New York.

The *Physician Associate Program* of *SUNY School of Allied Health Professions, Stony Brook, New York 11794*, offers a twenty-four-month program of "community medicine involvement, especially in disadvantaged and rural areas."

The first forty weeks are spent in classroom instruction, followed by a clinical period of sixty weeks. The core curriculum involves pathology, safety research, and research design; an interdisciplinary seminar and management concepts for allied health professionals are included in the second year. Clerkships are conducted in a hospital, clinic, and office setting.

Resident tuition is $1,150, nonresident $1,800. Books and equipment are budgeted at $500, with clinical transportation an item of $500.

Eligibility for junior-year college status is a requirement for admission. Courses in the biological sciences and mathematics *or* chemistry are prerequisites, with course work in psychology and sociology recommended. A year of direct patient-care experience is required. It may be met as orderly, nurse's aide, corpsman, emergency medical technician, or in another capacity. A B.S. degree in health sciences is earned, as well as certification as a physician's assistant.

The *Physician's Assistant Program* at *Touro College, 30 West 44 Street, New York, New York 10036,* is a twenty-four-month bachelor's degree program (in health sciences) which, while providing the training to serve in all settings of the health field, is also engaged in the preparation of men and women to offer skilled services to geriatric patients. The philosophy of the program firmly states that the availability of specially trained physician's assistants may often eliminate the need for hospitalization of the elderly, with its accompanying dislocation and cost.

Applicants should have completed two years of college and proved their competence in the sciences, mathematics, sociology, and psychology. A year of patient-care experience is also required. First-year courses include anatomy, chemistry, dentistry, immunology, medicine, microbiology, neurology, ophthalmology, public health, pediatrics, preventive medicine, radiology, rehabilitation medicine, surgery, and sociology of the aged. A second year of hospital rotations and experience in a doctor's office follows.

Estimated expenses cite tuition and fees at $3,600, with books and equipment $700.

A twenty-four-month program is offered by the *Physician's Assistant Program* of the *Bowman Gray School of Medicine, Winston-Salem, North Carolina 27103.*

Part of Wake Forest University, which offers a B.S. degree to those completing the program who have presented three years of college for admission, the program also awards a certificate to those who entered with only two years of college, who may then present their credentials to several other North Carolina institutions toward the baccalaureate. Six months of patient-care experience in a military or civilian setting is a requirement, as are both the SAT and the Mathematics Achievement Test, Level 1.

Tuition and fees for both residents and nonresidents total $3,600, with books and equipment $475.

The *Physician's Associate Program* of the *Duke University Medical Center, Durham, North Carolina 27710,* the nation's pioneer PA program, requires a minimum of one year of health-related experience and at least one acceptable college-level course in chemistry and one in biology. An outstanding high-school transcript and satisfactory SAT scores are necessary.

The twenty-four-month course of study is comprised of nine months in basic medical sciences followed by fifteen months of clinical work, the last ten weeks of which are spent in a primary care setting away from the medical center.

All pay a tuition fee of $3,830, with $575 needed for books and equipment. A certificate is offered students who complete the program but do not present sufficient undergraduate hours to qualify for the Bachelor of Health Sciences degree.

The *Physician Assisting Program* of the *Department of Allied Health, Cuyahoga Community College, Western Campus, Parma, Ohio 44130*, is a twenty-one-month course requiring high-school graduation, acceptable ACT scores, and two years of civilian or military health experience. The first year is wholly college-oriented. The next four quarters are spent in a variety of basic rotations, including internal medicine, peripheral vascular disease, cardiology, surgery, primary-care pediatrics, emergency room, dermatology, and experience in a primary-care center.

An associate's degree and certification are awarded. Tuition and fees total $425 for a county resident, $630 for other Ohio residents, and $1,000 for nonresidents. There are fees totaling $500.

ACT scores and high-school graduation are required for admission to the twenty-three-month *Physician's Assistant Program, Kettering College of Medical Arts, 3737 Southern Boulevard, Kettering, Ohio 45429*. Direct patient-contact experience of at least a year is mandatory, as is high-school graduation in a college-preparatory course. Considerable emphasis is given throughout the program on training to assist in a doctor's office.

An Associate in Science degree is earned. Tuition and fees are $2,066, with books and equipment estimated at $450.

A *Primary Care Physician Assistant Program* is offered by *Cincinnati Technical College, 3520 Central Parkway, Cincinnati, Ohio 45223*. The program leads to an associate degree and certification. It is of twenty-four months' duration.

The curriculum is "cooperative," each ten weeks of classroom course work followed by a corresponding ten-week clinical course. Courses include technical writing, communication skills, human relations, technical mathematics, sociology, obstetrics and gynecology, physics, chemistry, immunology, laboratory techniques, anatomy-physiology, and pathology.

High-school graduation and completion of an advanced chemistry course are admissions requirements. An associate degree and a certificate are awarded.

Tuition is $15 per credit for residents, $22 for nonresidents. Books and equipment total $500.

The *University of Oklahoma*'s *Health Sciences Center, Oklahoma City 73190*, has a twenty-four-month *Physician's Associate Program*, open to students who have had at least two years' experience in direct patient care and at least sixty credits from an accredited college or university.

After a ten-month didactic period, the clinical

program offers six weeks each of inpatient and outpatient medicine, general surgery, emergency medicine, and two elective clinics. An additional twelve weeks' primary-care training and an eight-week preceptorship conclude the course of study, which leads to a B.S. degree from the University of Oklahoma College of Medicine.

Tuition and fees total $1,780 for residents, $4,580 for nonresidents, with $600 needed for books and equipment.

The *Hahnemann Medical College and Hospital* of *Philadelphia, Pennsylvania 19102*, offers a twenty-one-month program open to high-school graduates who have had two years of "life experiences" at the time of making application. The experience might be educational and/or vocational; direct patient-contact experience is *not* a requirement. *Motivation*, however, is an important factor, with the admissions committee interested in those willing to serve in areas of greatest need, urban or rural.

The program consists of liberal arts, medical education courses, and a clinical practicum. In addition to twenty-four weeks of clinical experience in a variety of settings, each student spends six months in a preceptorship under the supervision of a primary-care physician.

Tuition and fees total $2,650, with books and equipment requiring another $220. The A.S. degree is awarded.

The *Physician's Assistant Program* of the *Texas Medical Center, Baylor College of Medicine, Houston,*

Texas 77025, is a twenty-four-month course described as innovative and open only to those who have completed two years of college, with courses in biology, chemistry, mathematics, humanities, and English. Experience in the health field is *not* essential.

The first nine-month period is spent in "concentrated medical sciences presented in a systems-oriented fashion." Clinical experiences follow, with students gaining competence in the treatment of all age groups. "Prior to completion . . . each student is expected to demonstrate his knowledge and ability through written, oral, and practical examinations." A B.S. degree is awarded.

Tuition and fees are $2,200, and another $400 is needed for books and equipment.

The *Physician's Assistant Program* is part of the *University of Texas School of Allied Health, 5323 Harry Hines Boulevard, Dallas 75235,* offering a twenty-seven-month course "designed to provide a firm base for the science and art of medicine." The senior year consists of mandatory and elective clinical rotations, with the latter planned to coalesce with the students' special interests and future plans.

Two years (sixty hours) of college are required; specific science and mathematics courses are indicated. A B.S. degree in health-care sciences and a certificate as assistant to primary-care physician are awarded.

Tuition and fees are $570 for residents, $3,990 for nonresidents. Another $425 is needed for books and equipment.

A very similar program is offered by the *University of Texas Medical Branch, Galveston 77550*. Fees are slightly higher.

The *Physician's Assistant Program* of the *Marshfield Clinic Foundation, Marshfield, Wisconsin 54449*, offers a twenty-four-month program individualized for each student. High-school graduation and three years of relevant experience in the health field are required. (RN licensure is accepted in place of such experience.)

The fifteen-month practicum utilizes a variety of settings, with the final two months spent with a physician preceptor in a small rural community in central or northern Wisconsin. The graduate is then awarded a certificate of completion by the Marshfield Clinic Foundation.

The student must budget $2,290 for tuition and fees if a nonresident, $1,080 if a resident of Wisconsin; $300 is indicated for books and equipment.

A *free* two-year program—one where you are actually *paid* to attend? Is there such a program outside the military services?

Indeed there is. It is the *Physician Assistant Training Program* of the *Medical Center for Federal Prisoners, Springfield, Missouri 65802*. Each student accepted is immediately placed on the Civil Service payroll at the GS-6 level for the first year and promoted to the GS-8 level the second year. ($10,370 and $12,763 respectively). Thus far, all who have completed the program have been offered jobs with the Bureau of Prisons starting at the GS-9 level ($14,097).

The student is charged no tuition or book fees. A certificate is awarded.

The first twelve months of the program involve lectures and clinical instruction at the Federal Prison Medical Center. The second year is conducted in another setting. The training, though well rounded, is geared to the training of individuals primarily interested in a career with the Bureau of Prisons Health Service Program.

The *Community Health Medic Program of Gallup, New Mexico 87301,* has been omitted because it is open only to persons with Native American Tribal affiliation and purports to train exclusively for work on Indian reservations.

INDEX

153

orders to PAs, 108
responsibilities for PA, 105
supervision, 108
value of PA to, 39
See also Doctor.
Physician Associate Program,
134
Physician's assistant, meaning
of, 40
Physician's Assistant in
Pathology Program, 131
Planning, value of career, 23
Poor people, doctor attitude
to, 87
Practice
limits of, 107
regulation of, 104
See also Work.
Preceptorships, financial aid
through, 77
Preparation for training, 24,
41, 96
Primary Care Associate Program, 133
Primary Care Physician Assistant Program, 148
Profession
development of, 90
future of, 111
Professional
limits, 76
status of PA, 37
Program, programs
applying to, 57
armed forces sponsorship
of, 126
federal support for, 38

after high school, direct,
127
MEDEX, 121
for medical specialization,
129
rejection from PA, 94
specialized training, 45
start of, 37
training, difficulty of, 25
training, length of, 120
various, 119
See also Education,
Training.
Psychiatric emergency, study
of, 69

Q
Quinnipiac College, 131

R
Records
medical, handling, 27, 29
medical, importance of, 13,
14
References, application, 59,
96
Regulation of PA practice, 104
Regulatory authority statutes,
104
Rejection from PA program,
94
applying after, 95
review of, 96
Respiratory therapist, 99
Responsibility
limits of PA, 107
physician, for PA, 105